'010

362.11 CON
Conlon, Patrick, 1944–
The essential hospital
handbook : how to be an
effective partner in a loved
one's care /

PALM BEACH COUNTY
LIBRARY SYSTEM
3650 SUMMIT BLVD.
WEST PALM BEACH, FLORIDA 33406

Praise for *The Essential Hospital Handbook: How to Be an Effective Partner in a Loved One's Care*

"This should be mandatory reading for both healthcare professionals and patients' families. We often forget how a patient's loved ones are an important component of healthcare delivery. In the current unbalanced healthcare system, we cannot afford to neglect the key insights provided by this invaluable resource."

—Thomas E. Stewart, MD, FRCPC, University of Toronto;
Physician-in-Chief, Mount Sinai Hospital;
and Associate Physician-in-Chief, University Health Network

"I will use and recommend Patrick Conlon's wonderful book. Patrick helped his loved one on the journey toward health, and now paves the way for a smoother journey for all patients."

—Jona Raasch, President, The Governance Institute

"The Essential Hospital Handbook will help to demystify the hospital experience for families and help them to manage their choices about care and treatment options."

—Mary Ferguson-Paré, RN, PhD, CHE,
Vice President, Professional Affairs,
and Chief Nurse Executive, University Health Network

Yale University Press Health & Wellness

A Yale University Press Health & Wellness book is an authoritative, accessible source of information on a health-related topic. It may provide guidance to help you lead a healthy life, examine your treatment options for a specific condition or disease, situate a healthcare issue in the context of your life as a whole, or address questions or concerns that linger after visits to your healthcare provider.

Joseph A. Abboud, M.D., and Soo Kim Abboud, M.D.,
No More Joint Pain

Thomas E. Brown, Ph.D.,
Attention Deficit Disorder: The Unfocused Mind in Children and Adults

Patrick Conlon,
The Essential Hospital Handbook:
How to Be an Effective Partner in a Loved One's Care

Richard C. Frank, M.D.,
Fighting Cancer with Knowledge and Hope:
A Guide for Patients, Families, and Health Care Providers

Marjorie Greenfield, M.D.,
The Working Woman's Pregnancy Book

Ruth H. Grobstein, M.D., Ph.D.,
The Breast Cancer Book: What You Need to Know to Make Informed Decisions

James W. Hicks, M.D.,
Fifty Signs of Mental Illness: A Guide to Understanding Mental Health

Steven L. Maskin, M.D.,
Reversing Dry Eye Syndrome:
Practical Ways to Improve Your Comfort, Vision, and Appearance

Mary Jane Minkin, M.D., and Carol V. Wright, Ph.D.,
A Woman's Guide to Menopause and Perimenopause

Mary Jane Minkin, M.D., and Carol V. Wright, Ph.D.,
A Woman's Guide to Sexual Health

Arthur W. Perry, M.D., F.A.C.S.,
Straight Talk about Cosmetic Surgery

Catherine M. Poole, with DuPont Guerry IV, M.D.,
Melanoma: Prevention, Detection, and Treatment, 2nd ed.

E. Fuller Torrey, M.D.,
Surviving Prostate Cancer: What You Need to Know to Make Informed Decisions

Barry L. Zaret, M.D., and Genell J. Subak-Sharpe, M.S.,
Heart Care for Life: Developing the Program That Works Best for You

The Essential Hospital Handbook

How to Be an Effective Partner in a Loved One's Care

PATRICK CONLON

Yale University Press   *New Haven and London*

The information and suggestions contained in this book are not intended to replace the services of your physician or caregiver. Because each person and each medical situation is unique, you should consult your own physician to get answers to your personal questions, to evaluate any symptoms you may have, or to receive suggestions for appropriate medications.

The author has attempted to make this book as accurate and up to date as possible, but it may nevertheless contain errors, omissions, or material that is out of date at the time you read it. Neither the author nor the publisher has any legal responsibility or liability for errors, omissions, out-of-date material, or the reader's application of the medical information or advice contained in this book.

Published with assistance from the Williams Memorial Publication Fund.

Copyright © 2009 by Patrick Conlon.
All rights reserved.
This book may not be reproduced, in whole or in part, including illustrations, in any form (beyond that copying permitted by Sections 107 and 108 of the U.S. Copyright Law and except by reviewers for the public press), without written permission from the publishers.

The right of Patrick Conlon to be identified as the Author of this work has been asserted by him.

Designed by Sonia L. Shannon.
Set in Bulmer type by The Composing Room of Michigan, Inc.
Printed in the United States of America.

Library of Congress Cataloging-in-Publication Data

Conlon, Patrick, 1944–
    The essential hospital handbook : how to be an effective partner in a loved one's care / Patrick Conlon.
        p. cm. — (Yale University Press health & wellness)
    Includes bibliographical references and index.
    ISBN 978-0-300-14575-5 (cloth : alk. paper) — ISBN 978-0-300-14576-2 (pbk. : alk. paper)
    1. Hospital care—Popular works.   2. Care of the sick—Popular works.   3. Consumer education—Popular works.   I. Title.
    RA965.6.C66 2009
    610—dc22

2008053908

A catalogue record for this book is available from the British Library.

This paper meets the requirements of ANSI/NISO Z39.48–1992 (Permanence of Paper).

10 9 8 7 6 5 4 3 2 1

*For Jim, as always—and for June Callwood (1924–2007),
who never excluded anyone*

Contents

Quick-Reference Sheets (following p. 342)
    Caregiver's Chart and Personal Journal
    Emergency Department Visit
    Living Will Legal Consultation
    Surgical Consultation
    Preoperative Assessment
    Questions for ICU Staff
    Handy Hospital Information
    Giving Updates to Family and Friends: Contact Information
    Caregiver Resources at the Hospital
    Surrogate Caregivers: Who, What, When
    Agenda for a Family Meeting/Conference
    Agenda for a Meeting to Plan Patient Discharge
    Home Preparation Checklist
    Presurgery Medications Checklist
    Medical/Surgical Follow-up Appointments
    Hospital Complaints Process
    Questions When Choosing a Hospice

Acknowledgments

Much like the kind of family-inclusive hospital care I seek to encourage, this book was energized by a belief in the power of collaboration. *The Essential Hospital Handbook* has emerged after years of informal but very helpful conversations with a large group of people I fondly call the Gang, borrowing a term that June Callwood used when she talked about righting wrongs. June, an old friend and prominent social activist who died in 2007, was responsible for starting more than fifty projects that have had positive and lasting social impact, but she always insisted that you first had to put a gang together before you could make significant change happen. She might have assembled a gang just like this if she had set her sights on overturning the conventional hospital-patient relationship.

But unlike June's gangs, this one has some members who have never met one another. They're spread all over the United States and Canada. Many are doctors and nurses with impressive credentials who have earned international reputations. Some run big hospitals or health-care organizations. Some help set national health-care policy. Some toil quietly in the background, making things better one patient at a time. Some lobby persistently for change.

All of them were available for even the wackiest of queries, and they were generous with their time and advice. And all of them demonstrate that special mix of compassion and commitment that seems to define people who can initiate positive change. They fiercely give a damn. They believe the best kind of health care heals the spirit as well as the body, and that the fundamental "we" of the community should be encouraged to gather for the challenge. I think June would have liked this gang.

As I name names, I'm going to leave off titles and degrees and affiliations and other impressive evidence of achievement. These people respond as human beings first and professionals second. They could be your neighbors. Count yourself lucky if they are.

With my deep thanks for their contributions to this book, meet the Gang: Roger Abbott, Andy Barrie, Donna-Marie Batty, Don Berwick, Donna Butt, Jenny Oey Chung, Tom Closson, Jim Conway, Katie Cronin-Wood, Mary Ferguson-Pare, Irene Ferko, Frances Flint, Frank Gavin, Jim Geiger, Elise Goldberg, Ed Hanada, Margaret Herridge, Kim Hitchings, Helen Hrdy, Mary Anne Huggins, Patricia Hynes, Beverly John, Bev Johnson, Noreen Kay, Norma Keen-Campbell, Diana Keung, the Kohl sisters, Stephen Lapinsky, Neil Lazar, Tina Leon-Garcia, Heather MacDonald, Toni Macdonald, Gail MacKean, Hume Martin, Kit Martin, Maryalice Mullally, Linda Nusdorfer, Harvey Picker, Jona Raasch, Frank Rosenberg, Nick Ruiter, Hilary Short, Tom Stewart, Gaetan Tardif, Sarah Telfer, Lieve Verhaeghe, Randy Wax, and Barbara Zuppa.

I also gratefully acknowledge the support of the Ontario Arts Council.

Introduction

"Would you like to ride along?" The question was almost casual. It was delivered with a smile. It seemed like a friendly afterthought.

It terrified me.

At that moment, my longtime partner lay unconscious a few feet away. He was now a bloated stranger, surrounded by tubes and wires and monitors and a big machine that apparently did all his breathing for him.

Jim had been admitted to the emergency room at the hospital two days before, short of breath and delusional, still claiming that he was getting over the flu. Within hours, he had been transferred to the intensive-care unit, where he was officially diagnosed with acute respiratory distress syndrome (ARDS), an uncommon and devastating illness with a very high mortality rate. ARDS doesn't stop with the lungs. Typically, it takes down the whole body—all the organs, one by one. It has been compared to a tsunami.

A doctor was asking the question. He had just admitted that his team had done all they could to save Jim but that Jim continued to lose ground. His lungs were not functioning anymore. "My gut tells me that he will die if he stays here," the doctor said. He saw only one remaining option, and it involved transferring Jim to a local hospital where some kind of investigational treatment—I didn't understand what—could be deployed in a last-ditch rescue attempt. "You should know there's a high risk that he could die in transit. Would you like to ride along?"

Some invitation. I hesitated, still in shock at the accelerating speed of the crisis, still wanting someone to wave a wand and make the bad news go away. I did not know then—perhaps fortunately—that the journey would be much longer than the brief run between hospitals.

I rode along in the passenger seat of a fat old ambulance, next to a pleasant driver who hummed off-key with the jazz on the dashboard radio. Two paramedics hovered over Jim in the back. He survived the journey, even improving slightly by the time we arrived at our destination, thirty miles away.

Jim went on to recover fully—after fifteen weeks of hospital care, a month of professional home nursing, and then nearly a year of physical rehabilitation. I was at his side for all of it, determined to be an active partner in his care and not just an anxious bystander. "We figured you weren't going away," said a charge nurse later, "so we decided to put you to work."

My tasks ranged from reading to Jim, attending to his basic grooming needs, and monitoring his physical and psychological responses while he sat in a chair for cardiovascular therapy to assisting with the dressing changes on two painful bedsores and suctioning bilious yellow stuff out of his lungs, from accompanying him to tests, supplying him with the music he liked, and advocating on his behalf for improvements in care or for clinical updates to helping him learn to speak and to eat and to walk all over again. I held him when he wept in frustration at the relentless struggle to rebuild his shattered body and spirit. I was just there, the one familiar person in a community of benign strangers rotating on and off shift.

And occasionally I reminded nurses and doctors, with respect, that they might be the experts on his illness but that I was the expert on him. Shift by shift over Jim's long stay, the staff moved from polite dismissal to grudging tolerance to acceptance of my presence. In the end they felt comfortable asking me how he was doing because they knew that I not only understood the question but knew that they needed to be aware of any changes in his mood or behavior that might be important when they reviewed their clinical assessments. The traditional circle of professionals around the hospital bed had now opened to include an ally—a feisty but well-informed and useful amateur.

One day a senior nurse stopped me on the way to Jim's recovery room. "I want you to know something," she said, with a veteran's weary bluntness. "He will get better sooner and go home quicker because you were here, because you were involved." That was all the validation I needed.

When he was finally discharged one snowy day in early April, he was handed over to me with a box of supplies and medications and a list of scribbled instructions. The staff were no longer wary. I had become a full partner in his care. They trusted that he would be in good hands. So did I, emerging from an intense learning experience that had taught me much about the complex ways humans strive to heal one another.

It was months before Jim and I were able to look back on the catastrophe and see the positives, among them the enjoyment of hospital care that acknowledged the value of a family member as an ally in recovery. What did we know? Before this crisis, neither of us had been near a hospital in twenty-five years. We assumed that all families were treated inclusively in the new millennium.

We were wrong. We came to realize that most families of hospital patients feel helpless and marginalized, outsiders in a system that relies exclusively on its own proficiency. They are left to languish in waiting rooms until permission to visit is granted. Worse, they are often treated as gatecrashers, reduced to pleading for time with their loved ones. With the professionals aligned against intrusion, standing guard like club bouncers, in most hospitals a we-know-best attitude prevails.

So Jim and I embarked on a campaign to promote hospital care that values active family participation. I wrote a series of columns for the *Toronto Star* that urged hospitals to treat families as an important care resource. *No Need to Trouble the Heart* (2007), my book about our hospital experience, has been used by medical-school teaching staff to show what can happen when the family is fully included in the care team. Jim and I have addressed several hundred hospital groups and international health-care conferences, never seeking invitations but responding to curiosity promoted by word of mouth. Everywhere we go, our message has been simple: families want in.

Most professionals in our audiences are open to the concept, although they don't know where to begin the process of integration.

Their training prepares them to be the sole experts. Others signal their skepticism with folded arms and peeks at their watches. They are not about to voluntarily share power.

Recent history seems to validate the skeptics. Until the 1950s, medical science could cure few serious health conditions. The time that nurses spent with patients was mainly to try to make them comfortable. Care was personal. But with the advent of gee-whiz drugs and technology, some of the humanity went out of medicine. Who had to worry about comforting or even understanding a patient when nearly every problem had a fix—a scalpel or radiation or a drug, or all three? Families were now expected to step back in awe and applaud the magic.

That scenario is starting to change. Internet-smart patients and families who once were intimidated by technological authority are now chasing answers to questions that would have been unspoken even ten years ago. A consumer society is growing accustomed to a level of service from hospitals that matches the customer service offered elsewhere, even though the relationship between patient and health-care provider is much too complex to be treated like a commercial transaction. Funding agencies and private donors are also prodding hospitals to tie patient satisfaction directly to their bottom lines and withholding critical financial support from facilities with poor patient-satisfaction scorecards. Some hospitals, eager to accommodate a market-driven economy, have even begun referring to patients as customers or clients. Either way, the them-us gap is closing. No one believes that time in a hospital has to be pleasant, but robbing the patient of therapeutic personal relationships for the sake of a clinical agenda is being openly challenged.

Including families in care is not an option in many parts of the world—it's mandatory. One of India's leading hospitals will not perform surgery unless a family member (or "attendant") agrees to sleep in the same room as the patient does for a night or two following the operation. A major Italian facility counts on families to provide and change every patient's bed linen—one more item off the hospital's list of patient-care chores. Health-care costs are escalating rapidly everywhere. Conceivably, hospitals in North America will also press families to take an active role in patient care. And maybe hospitals themselves will recognize that the best health care is collaborative.

The first shot across the bow of North American health-care arrogance was fired more than twenty years ago by a prominent Massachusetts physicist and inventor. The late Harvey Picker had spent a lot of time in hospitals as head of his family's successful X-ray business and also at the bedside of his wife, Jean, a former U.S. ambassador to the United Nations and a *Life Magazine* writer. Jean suffered from a chronic infection that required occasional hospitalization, and the couple saw firsthand how callously patients were treated by a system that professed to care. Many were abandoned on gurneys for hours, ignored by staff who shuffled around them. Patients were not people but cases—the diabetic in 29 or the brain tumor in 48 or the heart attack in 17. Waiting rooms were packed with anxious families who were made to feel as if they were in the way.

Harvey Picker set out to test a personal theory: that patients will do better if they are treated as human beings with acknowledged social and emotional needs. For the next seven years he worked alongside researchers at Harvard Medical School. After thousands of interviews with former patients and their families, the team eventually distilled its findings into eight guidelines designed to improve the hospital experience. Dubbed the Eight Dimensions of Patient-Centered Care, they have since become a guiding philosophy for hospitals who want to change the way they deliver care. One of the dimensions is "Involvement of Family and Friends."

The Picker approach has not been quick to catch on in North American hospitals, partly because many health-care professionals like, or at least feel comfortable with, the way things are. Despite emerging evidence that confirms Picker's findings (and the instincts of many professional caregivers), the idea that families can have supportive value at the hospital bedside is still being met with resistance. In certain specialties, however, family-inclusive care is already being practiced successfully. Most major children's hospitals in North America now welcome a high level of participation by parents, who know the patient better than they do. Hospices and palliative-care wards understand

that an active family presence can significantly improve the patient's final days. But many acute-care hospitals serving that vast patient population between birth and death have yet to get the message. For them,
chemistry and technology still rule.

That's why I set out to write the kind of book that I wish I could
have had in hand when Jim and I faced a serious health crisis for the first
time in decades. After one step into the hospital, I felt like a traveler
without a map, bumbling through the next frenetic stop on the tour
schedule. I needed basic information and strategy advice, fast. I needed
a quick look-up resource for all those baffling words. And I needed a
place to record information along the way—the course of treatment and
the tests, the victories as well as the setbacks, because recovery rarely
tracks in a straight line. All of those elements are here.

Frankly, this book is not for you if you are intimidated by authority
or if you are only comfortable with brief visits spent smiling at the patient and murmuring platitudes. This book is for families and friends
who believe that the more they know, the more they can help—for those
who are ready to roll up their sleeves and create a real care partnership.
Yes, if you offer to help, you could be rebuffed by harried staff too busy
to include you. Stand your ground politely but firmly. Remember—the
person in that bed is more important to you than to the staff, no matter
how sympathetic or skilled they are. The goal is to make home the next
stop on the patient's road to recovery. On that point at least, you and the
professionals can agree.

1
The Hospital
Nation of the Wounded

In a television interview a couple of years ago, the American commentator Richard Rodriguez talked about being admitted to a New York hospital as a cancer-surgery patient. "When they put that little identifying bracelet on your wrist," he said, "then you belong to a different nation. You belong to the nation of the wounded." Anyone who has always enjoyed good health might think Rodriguez was being melodramatic, but he was right. Every hospital is a foreign country, with its own language and rituals and shrines. That country's sole industry is hope.

Most patients are checked through the hospital border as naive and trusting pilgrims, willing to turn themselves over to strangers in the expectation that their failing bodies can be fixed. But there is a catch. In exchange for care, they are expected to surrender independence and endure feeling diminished and patronized. They are expected to be compliant with an agenda over which they have no real control. They will hear a bizarre language, eat boring food, learn to sleep surrounded by mysterious sounds and smells, relinquish personal privacy, and be shaken awake at 5:00 AM under the glare of lights so that someone can draw a blood sample. That's the deal.

If someone you love is hospitalized, it's important to have some understanding of the local culture. What's going on? Who are these people taking charge of my loved one's life? What are they saying? How do I encourage them to do what they do best without losing touch with the person I love while they are doing it?

Doctor's Orders

Hospitals may have earnest brochures and catchy slogans, but they are not warm and cuddly places. Most of them function like benevolent dictatorships, their natives conforming to a quasi-military system that runs on a rigid chain of command. Chiefs are at the top—the head doctor is the chief of staff, the top nurse is the chief nursing executive, and so on. Power is both valued and feared. Order, which is paramount, is secured by policies and procedures that are rarely challenged or even examined. Conduct is tightly regulated. Everyone displays rank with a uniform or a name tag, and even those flimsy and ubiquitous gowns for hospital patients are a uniform of sorts, adding peek-a-boo humiliation with rear ties that refuse to stay closed. The plastic bracelets are confirmation of subordinate status.

ASKED AND ANSWERED: Despite changing stereotypes, gender still weights health-care roles. In 2006, the American Medical Association reported that a majority of doctors in the United States were men: 72 percent. Nursing remains a predominantly female profession: fewer than 6 percent of nurses are men, according to a recent survey by the U.S. Department of Health and Human Services.

The military metaphors are pervasive. Care staff are called the front line. No matter how democratic the staff may appear, doctors in their emblematic white coats are conditioned to act like officers, and nurses like noncoms. In fact, it is still customary in some hospitals for nurses to rise respectfully whenever a doctor enters the room. Nurses sometimes call families "civilians" and converse among themselves about being on or off duty, or about tours of duty. Care itself is driven by formal orders (yes, "doctors' orders") that are followed obediently and on schedule by consulting the twenty-four-hour clock of the military, and it is delivered in hospital areas called units. The surgery prep room is called a holding area, and "war zone" is a familiar euphemism for the emergency department. In some hospitals it's common for emergency department staff to holler "incoming Scud!" as an alert to colleagues that ambulances are on the way with disaster casualties. And like combat pilots, they often use a thumbs-up gesture to signal readiness or affirmation.

But the military lingo finds its most companionable home in cancer treatment. There, newly diagnosed patients are frequently described as fighters—a way to raise their odds of survival and to comfort everyone around them.

Ever since U.S. president Richard Nixon signed the National Cancer Act in 1971 and publicly declared war on cancer, just about every cancer diagnosis has been followed by a declaration of war—and the proposed treatment for every patient is often expressed as a battle plan. The enemy is cancer, the commander is the oncologist, the soldier is the patient, the allies are the other members of the health-care team, and the weapons of choice are chemical, surgical, and nuclear. There is implicit pressure on the patient to support the myth that winning the war—defeating the cancer—is a matter of fighting courageously while suppressing any feelings of anxiety or uncertainty.

This strategy sustains the image of cancer treatment as a masculine, power-based, paternalistic, and violent campaign. It does not accommodate those patients who might feel pressed to keep struggling when opting out of treatment could be a better choice. Sometimes there is no evidence of medical benefit in continuing the fight.

The military theme even carries over into obituaries for cancer patients, whose surviving family members are captured by the rhetoric. The deceased is often saluted as a brave and noble fighter who finally had to surrender to—what?—a bunch of rogue cells with nothing on their teeny minds but self-replication.

Does the apparent rigidity of their organizational culture mean that hospitals are staffed exclusively by rule-worshipping automatons, driven only by clinical goals and imperatives imposed from above? Not at all. In fact, most care providers bring deep compassion to their work, and a sensitivity to suffering and loss that can be astonishing to witness. It's not unusual for staff at many hospitals to remain voluntarily past the end of their shifts simply to give comfort to patients and families in a crisis. There are hundreds of stories of extraordinary care, and most will never be documented in the professional medical journals because they cannot claim clinical significance. One memorable example from a few years ago involved nurses at a large urban Ontario hospital who were looking after a dying woman with a lifelong love of horses. She yearned to see her favorite horse one last time, but she was too frail to be moved from her room. The nurses arranged for the horse to be transported to the busy street adjoining the hospital, where it was led back and forth for a few minutes. Traffic stopped while the woman had a final view of her horse from her hospital window.

Some doctors and nurses have been known to weep openly with the family when a patient dies, and anecdotal reports of those episodes are perhaps partly responsible for sparking the current lively debate among professionals about the pros and cons of displaying emotion at the bedside. That the debate is occurring at all may provide evidence of an unvoiced collective desire to reconcile human and clinical ideals, projected against a traditional organizational belief that dispassionate military precision is essential for efficient delivery of clinical care. Proponents of a regimented management model argue that it helps staff deal with the high expectations that society imposes on health-care professionals by setting a framework in which care decisions and actions are both reasoned and swift.

The rank-sensitive nature of every hospital may not be immediately obvious to outsiders. It reveals itself at unexpected times, some of them even comical.

One day Jim and I were addressing a group of intensive-care doctors and nurses. The small conference room adjoining the intensive-care unit was jammed, and a man at the back with a camera on a tripod was videotaping the session for later viewing by staff who could not attend. While taking my turn at the podium I looked up and watched as the camera operator dropped slowly out of sight. The red light on his camera continued to blink, a beacon marking his descent. I announced that the camera operator had collapsed. No one reacted, including the doctors seated to either side of him. My God, I thought—the man could be dying. Why isn't anyone doing anything?

After a minute that felt like an hour, the senior doctor in the room rose and proceeded calmly toward the back of the room, a path for him opening automatically. He was immediately followed by two other doctors and then by a couple of nurses. The boss doctor made a quick appraisal, then stepped aside while the junior doctors improvised a gurney, finally rolling him away on a swivel chair, his head lolling alarmingly to one side. Again, no one else moved. The room was silent. The audience and I stared at each other, waiting for cues. A short time later, one of the junior doctors returned to announce that the camera operator had fainted: he was recovering from the flu and had not eaten anything all day. There were soft clucks of disapproval in the audience. The boss doctor nodded and sat down again, giving us a slight wave—a signal to continue. Afterward, no one spoke about the camera operator. The audience's response was rank-respectful throughout.

Issues of Control

Hospital codes of conduct also extend to visitors, those outsiders who are privately considered a potentially rowdy and capricious bunch but who are always publicly touted as valuable to patient recovery. Because maintaining order is paramount, visitors are expected to play by the house rules. Challenge to authority is not welcome here.

Visiting schedules are imposed at the discretion of each hospital, and they can vary widely. At one major Canadian facility, a family can visit any ward at any time of the day or night if the patient so wishes. At another large hospital a short drive away, visitors are restricted to four hours a day (5:00 to 9:00 PM), leaving the patient in the hands of well-intentioned aliens for the remaining twenty hours each day and begging an obvious question: Whose agenda is being served?

Many hospitals want to establish exclusive ownership of the patient by immediately assigning a specific and secondary role to visitors, no matter how intimate with the patient they may be. All post what they call visitor guidelines that cite patient welfare and comfort as the hospital's primary motivation. Some are patronizing in their admonitions. Others stop just short of outlawing gum chewing and running in the hallway. All seek to secure control. Here is a sampling that was culled from current guidelines posted by various North American hospitals:

- Being presentable helps the patient feel comfortable with you. Dress sensibly and wear footwear.

- Due to concerns about possible allergic reactions, scented flowers are not permitted in the hospital. All floral arrangements entering the building must come from approved local florists. The nursing desk will provide you with a list.

- Avoid prescribing your own remedies or giving medical advice. Doctors know what is best for their patients.

- Please leave promptly when the end of visiting hours is announced.

- Do not handle any hospital equipment or play with the bed controls. Doing so may harm the patient.

- Visitors are expected to withdraw immediately when a doctor enters the room to examine the patient.

- Children may visit but only with permission from the staff and only if they are accompanied by a responsible adult. Unruly behavior will not be tolerated.

- Always address the patient in a low and moderate tone. Be as cheerful as you can but avoid shouting and raucous behavior. This may disturb the patient as well as others.

- Please check with the staff before offering any food to the patient that was not prepared by the hospital. Most patients are on special diets and outside food is not always beneficial for them.

- Any visitor who persists in belligerent or disruptive behavior will be escorted from the hospital by security personnel. Smoking and consumption of alcoholic beverages are strictly forbidden on hospital premises.

- When a nurse needs to perform bedside tasks, such as bathing or moving the patient, please return to the family waiting room until you are summoned. A telephone near the entrance has been provided for that purpose.

ASKED AND ANSWERED: Many hospitals ban cell phones, claiming that they can interfere with sensitive medical equipment. However, in 2006 a Mayo Clinic research team activated two modern network-based cell phones from different makers in close proximity to 192 medical devices through 300 tests in 75 patient-care rooms. The four-month study concluded that "when cellular telephones are used in a normal way, no noticeable interference or interactions occurred with the medical devices."

While many hospitals have begun to relax their relationships with visitors, most still believe that even the most intimate of family members should not be invited to participate in the patient's direct medical care, or sleep in the same room through an overnight life-or-death crisis, or remain for bedside nursing procedures instead of submissively withdrawing, or question the purpose and validity of various tests. After all, the experts know what they are doing.

By these standards, a close family member will certainly not want to be present when a loved one's chest is being urgently cut open, perhaps splitting a rib or two, or when teeth are being accidentally dislodged to clear the breathing passage as expediently as possible because that loved one is in imminent danger of dying. In some hospitals, however, visitors are starting to be present in the room during routine as well as extraordinary medical procedures. The familiar scene of an exhausted doctor entering a waiting room and announcing solemnly to the worried family, "We did everything possible," is no longer good enough.

A Piece of the Action

If there is a symbolic battlefield where the fight for family inclusion will be won or lost, it is either the emergency department or the intensive-care unit. More than anywhere else in a hospital, both are places where death is a familiar presence.

Families want to stay close to a loved one when a crisis is at hand or when death could be imminent. Nurses and hospital chaplains started carrying that message to doctors about ten years ago, and the pressure for family inclusion is increasing. Modern hospitals have tended to sanitize death, to shield the public from its uglier aspects, but many families now opt to witness resuscitation attempts and to stay with dying relatives.

Supporters of the contentious idea claim that popular television shows like *ER* and *House* have already prepared the public for the potential gore and violence of resuscitation—and for the extreme tension that overtakes doctors when they are rushing to save a life. Chaplains especially also argue that allowing family members to watch could aid them in dealing with their grief, if all efforts fail and death results. In settings where the family is allowed to be present on an experimental case-by-case basis, nurses are reporting that family members who witness a resuscitation can help decide when to end efforts to revive the patient. The parent or spouse steps forward to tell the doctors that enough has been done and that it is time to stop the heroics.

ASKED AND ANSWERED: Abbreviating *emergency room* to ER is common in the United States despite efforts a few years ago to formally use the name ED (emergency department) because there is usually more than one room. The campaign failed, and critics reasoned that the new acronym was too closely associated with the widespread use of ED to describe erectile dysfunction. The huge success of the television show *ER* has also been blamed for public resistance. But even though *ER* is just as popular in Canada, the usual nickname there is *emerge*.

Family members have also been known to assist the resuscitation team by scolding the patient back to life. One wife commanded her husband to stop dying because his premature departure would be very inconvenient for the family. It worked.

Despite assertions by advocates that nearly half of North America's hospitals already allow some form of family presence at resuscitations (much of it unofficial or case by case), several studies reveal that nurses are starting to accept the practice but that many doctors continue to resist. The reasons vary. Some doctors believe that families might interfere with patient care and make rescue attempts even more stressful for everyone involved. Young medical residents, still nervously finding their feet in real-life medicine, often fear they will screw up—and be seen screwing up. All doctors are accustomed to power, and for many, the presence of the family feels like a revolutionary assault—an invasion of medicine's traditional inner sanctum. They may worry that medical decisions are no longer exclusively in their own hands.

Another factor seems to fuel resistance to family presence.

Western medicine is dominated by a push for machinelike perfection in the delivery of care. From the first day of training, medical students are told that errors are completely unacceptable. Although bonding with patients and their families is nice, every diagnosis must be considered, every allergy and previous medical problem must be reviewed, every X-ray must be perused, every drug dose must be accurate. In most operating rooms, every drop of blood is accounted for, and every move is logged. The bar is dauntingly high even before a resuscitation starts.

Most doctors want to believe that they have the training and skills to meet virtually any clinical challenge. They enjoy a natural high when they watch the flat line on a bedside heart monitor turn to peaks and valleys again: death averted. But when they have to deal with a failed resuscitation, when they have to formally pronounce a time of death after exploiting all of their knowledge and all of the tools at their command, then they are forced to confront their limits. They can share their feelings of dismay and frustration with sympathetic colleagues in the professional circle around the bed, which is normally closed to outsiders.

Adding an audience of strangers who weep over the dead body—tangible evidence of their failure—makes many doctors profoundly uncomfortable. They know they have done their best. Reason tells them that the family witnessed a full call on their proficiency and commitment. Reason also tells them that they will be spared the awful walk to the waiting room, with all eyes locked on them when they enter to deliver bad news. Still, many doctors choose exclusion. They believe that the process of failure, the exertion and sweat of desperate but ultimately futile moves, should be shuttered from public view. The end result is all that needs to be shared with grieving family members. It's less messy that way. It is also less human.

Doctors have come to count on the technical virtuosity that machines are capable of. Machines are more reliable than the patients they were invented to serve, more able to report the tiniest impulses of clinical response, and they reduce the odds of error. A persistent flat line on a monitor confirms that a patient is dead. Still, however superior the machines, we need doctors to help us understand what is happening and why. Many doctors appear not to understand that machinery can also help bring humanity back to medicine. Machines may make the call. But when they are switched off after resuscitation fails, a doctor's best work as a healer can begin.

In fairness to critics of family presence during moments of crisis and potential death, most families are not as ready for brutal reality as they think they are. Resuscitations can be gruesome. It is one thing to watch fake blood splattering the cubicle walls in a television show, with regular commercial breaks providing relief from the scripted agitation. It is another to witness real blood surge from the body of someone you love. A majority of resuscitation attempts depicted on television medical dramas appear to have happy outcomes, with doctors and nurses giving each other high fives when the patient's heart starts beating again. There are tears of happiness and relief all around when the patient blinks awake and asks for ice cream. The aftereffects are seldom negative.

But television dramas seldom mirror real life. In the late 1990s, a joint research team from Duke University Medical Center, the University of Chicago, and Durham VA Medical Center studied several popular medical shows—including *ER*—and the team's conclusions were published in the *New England Journal of Medicine*. Researchers reviewed sixty episodes that featured resuscitation attempts and calculated that nearly 80 percent of the patients survived. In a stark reality check, the team went on to report that the actual survival rate is closer to 15 percent and that surviving patients often suffer permanent brain damage or crippling neurological complications. Some of the television programs under scrutiny by the team may now be history, but current favorites like *House* and *Grey's Anatomy* appear to sustain viewers' apparent eagerness for quick fixes and happy endings. No matter how complex, most medical emergencies are usually wrapped up within the allotted sixty minutes. Minus commercials, of course.

So the controversial debate continues. On one side are nurses and chaplains, who say that they worry about the emotional needs of families. On the other side are doctors, who claim that their primary concern is the quality of clinical care. Overseeing both are hospital bureaucrats, who are wrestling with the implications for liability and anxious to protect the institution from potential lawsuits in the event of apparent errors or omissions.

The discussion is being driven by growing public calls for more transparency in health care. Families and friends of patients—potential patients themselves—want to know what goes on behind closed curtains. Watching a bunch of doctors and nurses struggling to save someone's life is about as transparent as it gets.

2

Emergency

Hurry Up and Wait

No one in the small Louisville City Hospital emergency waiting room had a clue about the crisis unfolding down the hall. An ambulance had just delivered a twenty-eight-year-old man who had lost a tavern brawl. He had four stab wounds in his heart and was bleeding profusely, but hospital staff were trained to do nothing in such cases except watch and wait—something Arnold Griswold was not good at. He broke the rules. This brilliant surgeon opened the patient's chest immediately, sutured the four holes, and shipped him off to recovery. The patient survived.

That was more than seventy years ago. Griswold was a pioneer in emergency medicine. Louisville City Hospital had opened the world's first trauma center in 1911, but Griswold was determined to expand its capabilities when he arrived as a young hotshot in 1932. He equipped Louisville police cars with medical supplies and trained officers in emergency care, making them the ancestors of today's paramedics. He helped establish Louisville's first blood bank and developed autotransfusion, the use of the patient's own blood during surgery. He invented a machine for treating fractures and then became an expert at fixing broken bones, perfecting the use of pins and walking casts. His decision to ignore conventional medical wisdom and operate on the stabbing victim was risky, but it paid off. Griswold could eventually claim the best survival rate for penetrating heart wounds in the United States.

But Griswold's quick-thinking improvisation, his necessary detour from less-critical cases competing for attention, may also partly explain why emergency wait-times are so long. Skills and technology have advanced since his day, but unpredictable calamity still hijacks orderly expectations. Too often, efforts to plan and schedule become meaningless. The waiting room fills with people leaning against walls or hunkered down in corners because all seats are taken.

Other reasons for the long waiting times are escalating public demands for urgent treatment, a shortage of skilled emergency doctors, and a scarcity of hospital beds to which critically ill or injured patients can be transferred after assessment by emergency staff. Insiders call these critical patients "bed blockers" because they occupy gurneys that cannot be used by other emergency patients until the patients are moved somewhere else in the hospital. Everything backs up.

The public demand for immediate care keeps rising. A survey by the U.S. government's Centers for Disease Control reveals that visits to American emergency departments totaled more than 119 million in 2006, up 32 percent over a decade. That works out to about 227 visits per minute, a record high that experts predict will soon be surpassed. Some patients will have minor aches that they think are life-threatening. Some will arrive in a panic because they are gasping for breath. Some will arrive with severed limbs, rushed on stretchers from a nearby train wreck or car accident. The ones whose limbs could possibly be reattached will obviously be treated first. The rest will wait an average three and a half hours to begin treatment if they are in the United States and just over two hours in Canada—but reports of eight-hour waits are not uncommon in either country, and there are horror stories in both countries of patients who die while waiting much longer to be assessed and treated.

While Canada's lower average waiting time may suggest superior efficiency, the reason probably has more to do with the difference in the way health-care delivery is managed in both countries. In 2007 the U.S. Census Bureau estimated that nearly 47 million Americans have no health insurance and therefore have no access to a family doctor. As a result, many of them are forced to resort to emergency departments for their primary health care. They know they will not be turned away: thanks to the Emergency Medical Treatment and Active Labor Act passed by Congress in 1986, the poor and the uninsured in the United States cannot be refused emergency treatment. But some American hospitals are now stepping around the law by closing their emergency departments, adding to the crush at those that remain open. Canada's publicly funded system eases the pressure on emergency departments somewhat by guaranteeing that everyone is entitled to access to health care (including a family doctor), but the much-reported grumbles about emergency wait-times continue.

Adding to the push to trim wait-times is a widespread professional belief that severely injured or ill patients treated within sixty minutes (the so-called golden hour) have the best chance of survival. This old theory is being challenged, but it still has a visceral hold on daily medical practice.

ASKED AND ANSWERED: The Institute of Medicine estimates that eighteen thousand adults in the United States die each year because they are uninsured and can't afford proper medical care. Many arrive in hospital emergency departments as a last resort, often much sicker than they would have been if they'd had access to primary and preventive care.

Another popular assumption in both countries is that dwindling emergency department resources are constantly stressed by people with inconsequential ailments. Whether they are too impatient to make an appointment with their family doctor or have another reason to head straight to the emergency department, some of their exploitive tactics are downright goofy. Anyone who has worked in an emergency department has an eye-rolling story to tell, like the one currently making the rounds about the woman with a broken fingernail who insisted on an ambulance ride to the hospital to have it repaired. Apocryphal? Maybe, but tales like that fuel accusations of service abuse.

Allegations of widespread abuse don't jibe with the facts, however. According to the U.S. government's Agency for Healthcare Research and Quality, sprains and strains, bruises and other superficial injuries, and abdominal pain are the top three reasons that most people seek emergency help. Chest pain is number four. Sore throats, infections, and other minor complaints (including broken fingernails) are way down the list.

Who Goes to the Emergency Department

Hospitals have to walk a careful line. They cannot actively discourage emergency department visits, because an apparently minor problem could be a symptom of a dangerous one. On the other hand, most would agree on the following general guidelines, provided by the American College of Emergency Physicians.

Who *Should* Go to the Emergency Department

Anyone, adult or child, who experiences:
    difficulty breathing
    chest or upper abdominal pain or pressure
    fainting, sudden dizziness, weakness
    changes in vision
    confusion or changes in mental status
    any sudden or severe pain
    uncontrolled bleeding
    severe or persistent vomiting or diarrhea
    coughing or vomiting blood
    suicidal feelings
    difficulty speaking
    shortness of breath
    unusual abdominal pain

A child who:
    has a persistent fever (more than 38.5 degrees centigrade/
        100.4 degrees Fahrenheit)
    has persistent vomiting and/or diarrhea
    will not eat or drink—particularly a child under five

Who Should *Not* Go to the Emergency Department

A family doctor or an urgent-care clinic would probably be more suitable to renew prescriptions or to treat people with these or similar conditions:

    minor burns or injuries

    sprains and strains

    coughs, colds, and sore throats

    ear infections

    fever or flu-like symptoms

    skin irritations (rashes)

    mild asthma

    chronic problems that need investigating

ASKED AND ANSWERED: There are about four thousand emergency departments in the United States and about eight hundred in Canada. With hospital amalgamations a strong trend in both countries, there are significantly fewer emergency departments than there were ten years ago.

This is the emergency department wish list. Real life, of course, has a minefield of unpleasant surprises. Emergency doctors see a wider range of conditions than any other medical specialists. In a typical week they will deal with:

    car accidents

    sports injuries

    broken bones and cuts from accidents and falls

    burns

    gunshot and knife wounds

    uncontrolled bleeding

    heart attacks, chest pain

    difficulty breathing, asthma attacks, pneumonia

    strokes, loss of function and/or numbness in arms or legs

    foreign objects lodged in various body cavities

loss of vision, hearing
unconsciousness
confusion, altered level of consciousness, fainting
suicidal or homicidal thoughts
drug overdoses
severe abdominal pain, persistent vomiting
food poisoning
blood when vomiting, coughing, urinating, or defecating
alcoholic blackouts
severe allergic reactions from insect bites, foods, or medications
complications from diseases, high fevers

When to Go to the Emergency Department

Competition for health-care dollars is fierce in both Canada and the United States, and hospitals rely heavily on community support. Gamely addressing the growing number of complaints about emergency wait-times, some American hospitals are taking unusual steps to reduce them. In a move reminiscent of pizza-delivery chains, one Kansas City, Missouri, hospital launched a "30-minute guarantee" program in 2007 to serve emergency patients, promising free movie passes if waits were longer. Not to be outdone, another Kansas City hospital immediately pledged that patients would enjoy door-to-doctor service within fifteen minutes of arrival. Other hospitals across the United States are now offering consolation prizes that they hope will lessen cranky feedback; unhappy patients receive such gifts as baseball tickets, prepaid gas cards, and meal passes, as well as a letter of apology from the hospital. One ambitious hospital emergency department even promises no waiting at all: it registers patients while they are being treated.

In Canada there are no prizes for waiting too long. All hospitals answer ultimately to political leaders, many of whom have turned wait-times into hot-button ballot issues, vowing solemnly that service will accelerate if they are elected. One Canadian province has even tabled a plan that would require each hospital to post its wait-times online in real time, which would allow emergency patients to consult the hospital's Web page for up-to-the minute information before setting out. Efforts to fix the problem on both sides of the border are starting to resemble a loony version of Wheel of Fortune.

ASKED AND ANSWERED: In 2002, Great Britain's Department of Health solved the wait-time problem by ordering emergency departments to assess and treat patients within four hours or face penalties. Currently, only 4 percent of all patients have to wait longer than that.

Politicians and health-care leaders have no control over certain variables. Wait-times are typically longer in big-city hospitals in either country simply because of heavier population density. Also, emergency staff at major urban hospitals routinely see many more victims of violent crimes and car accidents than do their nonurban colleagues, unpredictably increasing the pressure on already taxed resources. Wait-times can also vary by day of the week and by time. Weekends and Mondays are busiest. Peak hours are usually from 4:00 PM to 8:00 PM. Demand builds steadily through the day from 7:00 AM; the quietest periods often occur in the very early morning. Many emergency department staff also claim that the level of crowding and agitation in the waiting room increases when the moon is full.

Based on those statistics, you may want to schedule your next health crisis for 5:00 AM on, say, a Wednesday, somewhere in a small town safely past the time of a full moon. But crises tend to hijack the safe and the predictable. You may suddenly find yourself behind the wheel of a car, routines and plans tossed aside while you speed to the emergency department with someone you love squirming in discomfort beside you. Or—still not certain what happened or why but dreading the awful possibilities—you may be playing catch-up with an ambulance that carries an unconscious family member.

Life Interrupted: An Emergency Visit

Imagine this. It is 8:00 AM on a Monday. You are puttering around in the kitchen when your husband shows up at the breakfast table looking pale and shaky. He admits that the abdominal pain he mentioned last night has stayed with him. He figured it was just an attack of indigestion when he went to bed, but it got worse through the night and interrupted his sleep. The pain seems to be isolated in the lower right side of his abdomen. He is not usually a complainer, and now he has no interest in food, even juice or coffee, and does not finish the glass of water he accepted. You are starting to worry. You and he agree that you should call your regular doctor, but an answering machine announces that the office will not open for another hour. You know your husband hates hospitals, but you suggest that his best option is the emergency department. He is feeling too crummy to argue. You offer to go with him. He relaxes, just a little.

SMART MOVES: **Heading to the Hospital with a Patient**

- Bring a list of any medications (including herbal or homeopathic remedies) the patient has been taking. If a list is not immediately available, grab all prescription medicine bottles and supplies and dump them into a bag.
- Bring enough cash to cover parking, such incidentals as coffee and snacks—and phone calls if the hospital bans cell phones.
- Leave the patient's valuables—including watches, rings, and jewelry—at home, or plan to safeguard them yourself.
- Be ready to provide the name of the patient's family doctor and a brief health history (including known allergies), if possible, as well as proof of insurance (U.S.) or provincial health card (Canada).
- Bring a book or magazine to read unless you are fond of tattered old newspapers.
- Start thinking like a potential care partner, not just a spectator. A good first step: bring along this book—or tear out and bring

along the Emergency Department Visit quick-reference sheet at the back of this book—to make a record of the visit. The quick-reference sheet is also reproduced nearby in this chapter. (All the sheets appear both in the text for handy checking and at the back of the book as tear-out, take-along sheets. You are welcome to photocopy the sheets, too.)

Emergency departments function on a first-come, first-served basis, but serious cases automatically jump the line in a "worst first" priority ranking. At least they are supposed to. There are recurring stories of patients who died in the waiting room from various acute conditions because they were not seen quickly enough. In 2008, a homeless Winnipeg man waited thirty-four hours for treatment before he was eventually found dead.

Your husband would not be stalled in the waiting room if he had suffered a heart attack or a serious injury and had been transported by ambulance. Paramedics would have been in communication with emergency department personnel on route to the hospital; treatment may have already started in the ambulance.

He can walk. He's not the worst, so he's not first.

You and your husband have been fans of *ER*, but this is your first time in a real hospital emergency department, and you are startled by the noise and apparent confusion. Babies are crying. People are hugging themselves in obvious discomfort. A large family is gathered around a woman who is vomiting into a bowl. You hear coughing and sneezing, mixed with angry words quickly silenced. Every seat is taken, and people are standing in the corners and along the walls. Your husband is starting to perspire. You know that isn't a good sign.

Your first task is to help expedite things. The goal is to find out what is wrong with your husband and get medical attention as quickly as possible.

You and your husband approach the reception desk. He describes his pain, and you are both directed immediately to the triage nurse, a specialist whose job it is to assess the seriousness of your husband's complaint—and the urgency with which he should be seen by a doctor.

Emergency Department Visit
(Make as many photocopies as you need.)

Name of Patient and Relationship:

Hospital:

Address:

Date and Time of Arrival:

Patient Is Alert/Aware? Confused? Uncomfortable? (If yes, rate as Mild, Moderate, or Severe.)

Purpose of Visit

    Injury (cause, if known):

    Illness (symptoms):

Seen by Physician (name and time):

Tests Ordered:

Results:

Consulting Physician or Surgeon (name and time):

Final Diagnosis:

Held for Observation?

Projected Length of Stay:

Care Plan

    Treated in ER?   How:

    Admitted to Hospital?   Why and Where?

When Discharged from ER:

Prescriptions to Be Filled:

Recommended Home Care:

Symptoms to Watch For:

Recommended Follow-up Action:

Bring:

Proof of insurance (or health card)
Name of family doctor and contact information
List of patient's current medications (including herbal remedies and
    alternative therapies)
List of patient's known allergies

Leave at Home:

All of patient's valuables

Notes

ASKED AND ANSWERED: In 2007, Massachusetts' nonprofit Commonwealth Fund surveyed adult health-care experiences in seven countries, including the United States and Canada. It found that 34 percent of Americans want a major overhaul of the country's health-care system, compared with only 12 percent of Canadians. However, easier and quicker access to urgent care was high on the wish list among respondents in both countries.

The word *triage* is derived from the French word *trier,* meaning "to sort." A surgeon in Napoléon's army is widely credited with developing a simple system to swiftly evaluate battlefield casualties. Those with the most serious injuries would be treated or evacuated first. Modern emergency departments have adapted and improved that system. Although some still sort patients into three basic categories (Emergent, Urgent, and Stable), many now rate patients according to five different levels, which is considered more efficient. Level 1 is the most critical.

A typical example of this improved approach to patient assessment is the Canadian Triage and Acuity Scale (CTAS).

Level 1—RESUSCITATION: The patient's condition threatens life or limb and requires immediate, aggressive intervention. Examples: heart attack, major trauma, severe head injury, amputation.

Level 2—EMERGENT: The patient's condition presents a potential threat to life or limb and requires rapid intervention. Examples: severe difficulty breathing (due to asthma, allergic reaction, etc.), unconsciousness, severe bleeding.

Level 3—URGENT: The patient's condition could potentially progress to a serious problem requiring emergency intervention. Examples: head injury, deep cut, chest pain (unrelated to a known heart problem), foreign bodies in the eyes, evidence of a serious infection.

Level 4—LESS URGENT: The patient's condition could be related to age and/or distress, resulting in the potential of deterioration or complications. Examples: possible fracture or sprain, back
pain, skin or wound infection, serious headaches.

Level 5—NON URGENT: The patient's condition may be acute
but non-urgent, including evidence of a chronic problem with or
without evidence of deterioration. Examples: colds or flu, minor
cuts or bumps, bites, sore throat, sinus problems, dressing changes,
prescription renewals.

The CTAS system has been in widespread use across Canada since
the late 1990s, and variations are now found all over the world. The
United States remains an exception. American hospitals have been
slow to revise their emergency-assessment strategies, and a majority
still use the older three-level system. But movement toward establishing a standardized global five-level system is picking up.

The triage nurse will not have any interest in you or your anxiety.
Don't take it personally. She is trained to assess patients quickly, and
your husband needs all of her attention. Her job is to quiz him carefully
(examples: "Are you in pain?" "Where does it hurt?" "When did it
start?") and decide how urgent the problem is. She may also give a
quick physical exam to check such basics as pulse rate, respiratory rate,
and blood pressure. She takes a brief health history and asks about current medications of any kind that your husband is taking, as well as any
allergies he may have. She also checks his temperature. It is 101 degrees
Fahrenheit, confirming your suspicion that he is running a fever.

A nurse cannot officially diagnose a condition—only a doctor can
do that. Instead, the triage nurse's primary responsibility is to identify
and report each patient's "chief complaint." That formal term is entered in the patient's medical record. Knowing the chief complaint allows the doctor to proceed from a baseline of observed signs and reported symptoms. Your husband's chief complaint is severe abdominal
pain. If you ask the triage nurse, she might reveal that he could have appendicitis, based on the location of his pain and the fever, but that diagnosis is subject to confirmation by the doctor.

When the triage nurse finishes, ask her what your husband's assessment level is. If he probably has appendicitis and the hospital is using the CTAS scale, she will probably say that it is Level 3—Urgent because a burst appendix might be a looming risk. This could be useful information, not only because it tells you immediately how serious the problem appears to be but also because it provides an indication of the length of time you can expect to wait for a doctor's attention.

ASKED AND ANSWERED: To keep traffic flowing, many hospitals have introduced a fast-track system for treating emergency patients with minor complaints like cuts and bruises. They are seen and then treated quickly by a nurse and don't need to see a doctor. In Canada, about 70 percent of emergency patients tended this way need no further care and are able to leave promptly.

Your next stop is the registration desk, rarely seen on *ER* because paperwork lacks heart-pounding drama. The clerk will want your husband's vital statistics, his health insurance card, and the name of his regular doctor. This is the start of developing an official medical record so that all your husband's data, as well as any tests and procedures, can be entered on one chart. If applicable, a bill will also be generated from this information.

Then you and your husband return to the waiting room. The crowd is still large, but you find a couple of empty seats. You sit and wait. The hard part begins.

SMART MOVES: **Waiting**

- Find a nearby source of fresh water in case the patient gets thirsty.
- If a snack bar is close by, buy some plain crackers for the patient in case of hunger, but check at the reception desk before feeding anything to the patient.
- Find the nearest payphone (or step outside with a cell phone) to let concerned family members know what is going on.

- If the wait for attention seems long and the patient is growing more uncomfortable, alert the staff at the desk. Emphasize that you are concerned about the patient; do not emphasize your own inconvenience.
- Indicate your wish to remain with the patient for the doctor's examination in order to relieve the patient's stress and discomfort in an unfamiliar environment. Expect permission to be granted if you are requesting this for the sake of the patient.
- Update the Emergency Department Visit quick-reference sheet. Continue to update it when you have other opportunities. Reviewing it now—perhaps your first opportunity—will also give you an idea of what to expect and what to ask during the rest of your visit.

Despite the crowd in the waiting room, you and your husband don't have to wait long before you are called. You are grateful for the speed, but you also wonder if his condition is more serious than you feared.

The Examination Room

You are both brought to the exam room, a cramped cubicle around a corner and away from the waiting room. On the way, your husband threw up in the first washroom he found—which could be further evidence of appendicitis. An emergency department nurse meets him and obtains more detailed information about him. The nurse gets him settled into a patient gown so that he can be examined properly. She requests a urine sample.

Once the nurse has left, there is another wait before the doctor arrives. Emergency department doctors always seem to be in a hurry, and this one is no exception. He comes bustling in and has a quick look at the accumulated notes about your husband.

Then he and your husband exchange a couple of comments about the game they both watched on television last night. Your husband is nearly doubled over in pain, but he can still work up enthusiasm for a bottom-of-the-ninth home run. The doctor is busy, but he can spend a few seconds on baseball—and establishing rapport with the patient.

The doctor extracts a more detailed medical history from your husband and does a more thorough physical exam than the nurse did. He is moving toward a "differential diagnosis" by weighing one probable cause against others that might account for your husband's pain and its specific location. He already has the result of your husband's urinalysis. It is normal, which means that he can rule out a urinary tract infection, which can sometimes mimic appendicitis. But the doctor admits to both of you that appendicitis can be tricky to diagnose. He wants to order a complete set of blood tests.

Samples of your husband's blood are drawn and placed in tubes, each with its own additive depending on the test being performed.

> *A purple-top tube is used for a complete blood count (CBC). A CBC measures:*
>> the adequacy of his red blood cells, to see if he is anemic
>> the number and type of white blood cells (WBCs), to determine if an infection is present
>> the number of platelets (platelets are a blood component necessary for clotting)
>
> *A red-top tube is used to test the serum, the liquid or noncellular half of the blood.*
>
> *A blue-top tube is used to test the blood's clotting ability.*

You will have to wait while the samples are shipped to the lab for analysis, and you can guess that the doctor is not going to hang around. Sure enough, with a quick apology he races off to see another patient. Your husband is now squirming on the gurney, trying to find a comfortable position, and you check your watch every few minutes. Pending a confirmed diagnosis, he cannot be given anything to ease his discomfort. All you can do is be with him, and you try to distract him by chatting about your family.

Finally the doctor returns with the blood-test results. They indicate an elevated WBC count. This is a sign of a bacterial infection, and bacterial infections are commonly associated with appendicitis. All other results are within normal range.

The doctor is quite certain by now that your husband has acute appendicitis, and he tells you that he is going to bring a surgeon in to assess him for surgery. He shrugs sympathetically when you ask him how long it will take for a surgeon to arrive: another wait. Your husband has not said much, but he announces that he is getting hungry. The doctor shakes his head. He tells your husband not to eat or drink anything because he is possibly facing immediate surgery. An empty stomach can prevent potential complications from the anesthetic. With that, the doctor vanishes again.

Tools of the Trade

Time passes. Your husband has now been given antibiotics to deal with the infection and something to relieve the pain, thanks to a nurse acting on direction from the doctor. He dozes off. You find yourself looking around and wondering about this place of hurry-up-and-wait medicine.

A nurse pops in to make sure everything is okay. She checks your husband briefly. In a whisper, motivated more by boredom than by interest, you ask her about a piece of equipment parked in the corner and are told that it is a back-up ventilator, also called a respirator (used to administer oxygen). The nurse checks her watch and offers to take you on a quick tour. You accept, glad to take a short break.

Like many emergency departments, this one has been subdivided into separate areas so that patients can be treated efficiently. Various cubicles are enclosed only by curtains. Both you and the nurse are careful to avoid invading the privacy of patients you pass, but the vivid sounds of grief and discomfort in the cubicles are hard to ignore. Besides the curtained cubicles, there are a pediatric area, a chest-pain area, a trauma center (usually for severely injured patients), and an observation unit (for patients who do not require immediate hospital admission but who might require prolonged treatment or a lot of diagnostic tests). The place is a maze.

The department is stocked with a huge array of equipment, including devices with weird shapes and names. All of them have specific purposes. Some of them beep and blink. The nurse shows you typical equipment.

Stethoscope

A stethoscope, the nurse tells you, is an essential diagnostic tool for monitoring the heart and listening for abnormal sounds. One heart sound easily heard with a stethoscope is a heart murmur—which could be a sign of an abnormal heart valve. Heart sounds are also used to help a doctor or nurse determine the rhythm of the heart. A sound like a friction rub could be a sign of pericarditis (inflammation around the heart). Irregular or rapid heart sounds could be a sign of heart failure.

A stethoscope is also used to listen to the lungs. A doctor can diagnose various conditions like pneumonia, asthma, and pneumothorax (a collapsed lung) just by listening.

ASKED AND ANSWERED: Though now as universal in hospitals as the white coat, the stethoscope endured a rocky introduction to medical practice. From the *London Times,* 1834: "That it will ever come into general use, notwithstanding its value, is extremely doubtful because its beneficial application requires much time and gives a good bit of trouble, both to the patient and the practitioner, because its hue and character are foreign and opposed to all our habits and associations."

A doctor or a nurse can take a patient's blood pressure (BP) by using the stethoscope to listen to the flow of blood through the arteries. A BP reading is obtained when a BP cuff is wrapped around the arm and inflated to a pressure high enough to stop the flow of blood to the large artery on the inside of the elbow. A stethoscope is placed over this artery below the cuff, and air is slowly let out of the cuff. Blood flow starts when the pressure in the cuff becomes lower than the pressure in the artery. This creates a sound that can be heard with the stethoscope. The pressure on the BP gauge is the upper number in a BP reading. The lower number is the pressure at which the artery is no longer compressed and the sound stops. A normal BP is 120 for the upper number (systolic BP) and 80 for the lower number (diastolic BP). Any significant deviation from a 120 over 80 reading could be cause for concern. Evidence of high blood pressure (an upper number much higher than 120) will draw immediate attention from a doctor.

Cardiac Monitor

A cardiac monitor gives a visual display of the rhythm of the heart. This is vital information, particularly during a heart attack, when a patient can suddenly develop a lethal (life-threatening) cardiac rhythm. The patient is connected to the monitor by three sticky patches on the chest, which are attached by wires to the monitor. Cardiac monitors are set to sound an alarm if the heart rate goes above or below a predetermined number. Some monitors also have an automatic blood pressure cuff as well as a pulse oximeter, which measures the oxygen saturation of the blood.

Suture Tray

This tray holds the sterile equipment needed to place sutures (stitches) in a patient with a laceration: a needle holder (the instrument that holds the needle containing the suture material), forceps (used to hold the lacerated tissue together while it is being stitched), sterile towels (used to drape off the nonsterile areas that are not being repaired), scissors, and small bowls (to hold antiseptic solutions).

Orthopedic Equipment

Most emergency departments have a generous supply of orthopedic devices to deal with sprains, breaks, and fractures. The devices include plaster and/or fiberglass to make splints and casts. There are also pre-made splints for specific joints, such as knee immobilizers, aluminum finger splints, Velcro wrist splints, shoulder slings, air splints (for ankles), and cervical collars, as well as cast cutters to use when a cast has become too tight.

Crash Cart

The nurse explains that cardiac arrest (when the heart stops beating) is high on the list of conditions seen by any emergency department. People often arrive complaining of chest pain and go into cardiac arrest while they are waiting—or even while they are being assessed. Some complain of another condition entirely, but that condition can exert extraordinary stress on the heart, putting the patient in danger.

A crash cart is a cabinet on wheels with equipment and supplies used by doctors and nurses when a cardiac arrest occurs and immediate life-saving measures are needed. About the size of an old-fashioned washing machine, it has labeled drawers and compartments for quick retrieval of anything needed. Here are some of the items found on a typical crash cart.

Defibrillator—An electrical device with two paddles that are placed on the chest to discharge electricity through the heart when a lethal rhythm is evident. The aim is to shock the heart back to normal. The most common lethal rhythms present during a cardiac arrest are:

VENTRICULAR FIBRILLATION: The ventricle (main chamber of the heart) is twitching, causing a rapid, unsynchronized, and uncoordinated heartbeat

VENTRICULAR TACHYCARDIA: The ventricle is contracting rapidly, producing insufficient blood flow out of the heart

ASYSTOLE: The heart has stopped beating

PULSELESS ELECTRICAL ACTIVITY (PEA): The heart rhythm should be producing a pulse, but it isn't

BRADYCARDIA: The heart is beating so slowly that not enough blood is pumped out of it

Cardiac drugs—During a cardiac arrest, certain potent drugs are required to restart the heart or return it to a more stable rhythm. Some of the drugs used are:

EPINEPHRINE: Used in cases of ventricular fibrillation, pulseless ventricular tachycardia, asystole, PEA, and sometimes bradycardia

ATROPINE: Used in cases of asystole, bradycardia, and sometimes PEA

LIDOCAINE: Used in cases of ventricular fibrillation and ventricular tachycardia

Endotracheal intubation equipment—Endotracheal intubation is the procedure of placing a tube into someone's trachea (windpipe) when that person stops breathing or is not breathing adequately. The tube allows artificial respiration equipment to take over the job of breathing. The intubation package includes tubes of different sizes and a laryngoscope (a flexible tube with a light for examination of the larynx).

Central vein catheters—These catheters (thin flexible tubes) are placed in the large central veins (located near the heart) so that medications and fluids can reach the heart and other important organs quickly.

The nurse tells you that all kinds of other equipment are used in an emergency department, including the chest-tube tray, which holds the equipment needed to insert a chest tube (a tube placed between the ribs and the lung to re-expand a collapsed lung), and an ear, nose, and throat tray, which holds specialized equipment deployed most commonly to handle nosebleeds and to remove foreign bodies. But she has given you the highlights, and you admit that you've now seen more of an emergency department than you ever wanted to. She laughs and then glances at her pager before disappearing around a corner.

Second Opinion, First Smile

After two hours of waiting, the surgeon arrives. She performs her own physical exam of your husband and reviews all his lab data as well the notations from the doctor who saw him. She mentally catalogs his symptoms and test results—pain and tenderness in the lower right abdomen, vomiting, low-grade fever, and elevated WBC count. She and the emergency doctor agree: all the signs point to acute appendicitis. The medical response: removal of the appendix in a surgical procedure called an appendectomy, which is always treated as emergency surgery. The surgeon explains what is involved, including the risks and benefits. Your husband is asked to sign a consent form giving permission to operate. The surgeon tells you that your husband will be admitted to the hospital immediately and that surgery will take place later in the day. She does not foresee any complications and describes the operation as routine.

It is now just past 2:00 PM. For the first time in six hours, you can allow yourself to take a deep breath. For the first time since last night, your husband smiles. The agonizing pain will soon be over.

3
The Living Will
Saying Yes or No to Medical Intervention

Remember Terri Schiavo? She was a young woman who collapsed in her Florida home one day in 1990. Paramedics could not revive her. In addition to heart and respiratory failure, she suffered irreversible brain damage and became dependent on a feeding tube for survival. Her eventual diagnosis was persistent vegetative state (PVS), a condition in which there appear to be sleep-wake cycles but there is no evidence of conscious thinking during the "awake" periods.

In 1998 her husband (who was also her legal guardian) petitioned a local court for permission to have her feeding tube removed, knowing that she would certainly die but convinced that she would want her severely diminished life to end. Her parents vigorously opposed him, arguing that she was still cognizant and that withholding basic nourishment would constitute "judicial murder." The court agreed with her husband and ruled that Schiavo would not wish to continue life-prolonging measures. Permission to remove the tube was granted. But Schiavo's family appealed the decision before any action could be taken, and launched a high-profile legal battle that raged up the ladder through various courts for seven years, eventually involving both Congress and the White House. The family finally exhausted all legal options, and Terri Schiavo's feeding tube was removed on March 18, 2005. She died thirteen days later. She had been institutionalized for more than fifteen years and left a legacy of heartbreak and anger. Her husband was with her when she died. Her parents were not allowed into the room until he had left.

Ultimately the legal system gave weight to medical opinion about Schiavo's prospects, in conjunction with her husband's steadfast claims that he knew what she would have wanted. Her parents' insistence that she recognized them even in her so-called vegetative state and that she clearly wanted to live did not prevail.

Would Terri Schiavo have wanted this anguished strife for the people she loved? Probably not. The decision might have been easier on everyone if her wishes had been documented. That's why living wills and other advance directives make sense. They speak for those who can no longer speak for themselves.

Not so long ago, a person in Terri Schiavo's minimally responsive state would not have survived more than a few days. Advanced life-support technology did not exist. Keeping someone alive using artificial means was not an option. Most of us are glad that it is now available, especially if we see it as a temporary measure that could lead to the restoration of health. But it could also be undesirable—it may only prolong the process of dying. Or the patient might survive but face a very unsatisfying kind of life—unable to see, speak, hear, or move, for example. Under U.S. and Canadian law, everyone has the right to decide whether to start, continue, or withdraw life support for himself or herself. And as long as a patient is mentally competent, that patient can be consulted about what he or she prefers.

But matters can grow very complicated if a patient has lost the ability to communicate—which is why a living will (also called an advance directive) can be a useful ally if you are a family member trying to convey your interpretation of the patient's desires to a group of skilled and compassionate strangers who are committed to prolonging life, not to ending it. Without a living will, treatment using any means available to maintain the patient's life would probably continue, even over the objections of family members. For a living will to prevail in whatever those circumstances might be, time and careful thought are required of the person crafting it. Just filling in blanks will not do. If the document is legally challenged, it must pass muster in courts that demand clear and convincing evidence that it accurately reflects the patient's wishes.

Many hospitals now routinely ask patients being admitted if they have a living will. Some even make it a requirement and provide their own generic version for immediate signature, turning up the pressure in a situation already overlaid with anxiety. From their perspective, they want to know before treatment starts how far they are empowered to go to save a life.

The question is easily resolved if the loved one you are accompanying to the hospital is fully conscious and capable of making decisions. Paperwork and another few minutes at the admissions desk take care of the matter. But how would you respond in a medical emergency if your loved one is sliding into a coma and you are left guessing what she or he might want done when organs begin to fail: taking heroic measures or letting nature take its course?

Even if every family member is healthy, one of your first tasks as a family caregiver should be to encourage each one to have a living will. Maybe this is an insurance policy that might never be needed. Maybe you can bring the rest of the family around to the unsettling idea of needing a living will by being the first to prepare one.

Anyone over eighteen can prepare a living will, and you don't have to consult a lawyer. All you do is spell out how you would like to be cared for if you are unable to communicate what you want. Most jurisdictions where living wills have legal standing will provide forms; you can usually download copies from the appropriate government Web sites, all of them consistent with individual state or provincial standards. But a lawyer can help customize one that fits your specific needs and work with you to produce a document that addresses all possible issues. It might be portable between states or provinces, or even between countries.

ASKED AND ANSWERED: Living wills, whatever they are called in a given jurisdiction, have legal standing in forty-five U.S. states and all ten Canadian provinces.

"Some Conditions Apply"

Some people know right now that they will never want a certain kind of treatment under any circumstances, but this attitude is rare. Many medical conditions are reversible, and most of us would agree that even an unpleasant treatment could be tolerated for a short time if there are solid grounds for hope. More commonly, people have conditional wishes. They want to receive or refuse specific treatments depending on the circumstances, and they want control over some of the variables that might trigger their requests.

Generally, there are two types of situations in which a carefully prepared living will could be extremely important. The first is a terminal illness. The second is permanent disability.

When death is expected in a short time, people with a terminal illness often fear treatment that extends life without restoring their desired quality of life. Those who believe just being alive is all the quality of life they need may accept that kind of treatment. Others reject the idea of being alive while sliding relentlessly toward imminent death. If you lose the ability to communicate, your doctors may assume that you want your life extended as long as possible. If you prefer a shorter but more comfortable life during a terminal illness, you can request it. Most living wills can address the issues of terminal illness, and most doctors readily respect the wishes expressed about terminal care.

But a lot of living wills fail to address the other major fear that most people have: permanent disability resulting from an illness or an injury. It is harder to reach consensus about permanent disability for two reasons.

The first is that doctors and other health-care providers may attempt to impose their own value systems in a particular case. Although they may agree to withhold attempts to prolong life in a case of terminal illness, they may vigorously resist withholding treatment for a chronic and debilitating condition.

The second reason is that the range of chronic impairments is so great that people widely disagree about what constitutes an intolerable situation. Some may dread a stroke that leaves them unable to communicate. Others fear permanent dependency on others or the impaired thinking resulting from dementia or Alzheimer's. Since the circum-stances that trigger the application of a living will to chronic illness are different for each individual, each of us has to decide in advance what circumstances, if any, we would not wish to endure. The triggering cir-cumstances need to be defined as specifically as possible in terms of three primary factors: type, severity, and permanence or irreversibility. Terms like "loss of dignity" or "impaired ability to communicate" should be avoided because they can mean different things to different people. For instance, a minor stroke causing slurred speech may not be what some people mean by "impaired ability to communicate."

How do you determine what is permanent or irreversible? In most cases, the best anyone can do is to observe the patient for a period of time. Failure to improve over the short run may indicate a poor progno-sis in certain types of cases. A good example is brain damage due to lack of oxygen after cardiac arrest or a stroke. The longer a patient is uncon-scious, the less likely it is that full capacity will be regained. But who will regain full capacity and who will remain in a severely impaired state is impossible to predict immediately. Most people who will improve sig-nificantly show signs of progress in the first few days and generally within the first two weeks. It is usually reasonable to observe a patient for this length of time. Someone who does not wake up after two weeks is more likely to remain in a coma or a persistent vegetative state like Terri Schiavo, despite the rare exceptions that get a lot of publicity.

Fortunately, this kind of predictor (waiting and watching) supports the need to be specific in the living will. You can pick a time limit and state it in the document. Your doctor can even give you general progno-sis guidelines to help individualize your requests. A time limit (even a long one) protects against permanent maintenance in an undesirable state because a time limit is an unequivocal instruction. You can still use words like *permanent, irreversible,* and *hopeless,* but be aware that these alone are hard to interpret if you haven't set time limits. You may wish to be specific, setting a time limit like two weeks or thirty days dur-ing which there has been no clinical change in your condition.

There is something else you should consider while you're mulling over your options.

Many people decide to create a living will after witnessing the medical ordeal of a friend or relative. The experience might have made them wary and unsettled. Or they remember the media coverage of the Terri Schiavo case and vow not to have their own compromised lives extend for years and then end that way. Such events might stir you to add emphasis and weight to your own living will statements. Although no two sets of circumstances are identical, your real-life experience has given you familiarity with at least one that you wish to avoid. But you should not confine your comments to just the one set of circumstances unless you want to limit the application of your living will to exactly that and no other.

As you sort out your thoughts and understandable uncertainties about what you want your living will to express, remember to be specific about the types of treatment you want withheld. Many off-the-shelf living wills, the kind you can buy online, optionally instruct doctors to withhold "extraordinary care" or "life-sustaining" or "life-prolonging" treatments. In some cases, you are required only to check off the box to the right on the form. Just know that generalizations like these might be open to interpretation. They're less likely to be respected in the hospital or in court than those that are not ambiguous.

ASKED AND ANSWERED: Surveys suggest that most people are in favor of some form of living will. But a 2005 Gallup Poll revealed that only 40 percent of Americans actually have one. Of that group, 59 percent lack a living will that clearly dictates how little or how much medical intervention they would prefer.

The line between ordinary and extraordinary care used to be obvious, but it is shifting. Complex, expensive high-tech treatments are now common—they can hardly be called extraordinary anymore. On the other hand, people often object to the use of a simple, inexpensive measure to maintain life—a feeding tube, for instance. And many treatments can be considered life-sustaining even though their withdrawal may not result in immediate death. The real reasons that people reject certain treatments may be the circumstances surrounding their use. A ventilator (respirator) might be acceptable during treatment for pneumonia, but not necessarily after two weeks of observation following a cardiac arrest. Dialysis might be appropriate for a patient recovering from a major infection, but not necessarily for a patient wasting away from terminal cancer.

Here's a quick guide to some of the most common medical interventions.

TREATMENT: Cardiopulmonary resuscitation (CPR)

PURPOSE: To restart the heart and breathing

WHEN USED: Following a major heart attack

BENEFITS: Can often revive young, healthy people.

LIMITATIONS: Not as effective in older adults and the terminally ill. May prolong life only temporarily.

WHAT HAPPENS IF NOT USED: Coma leading to death within five to ten minutes.

TREATMENT: A ventilator

PURPOSE: To assist with breathing or completely take over breathing

WHEN USED: When an injury or illness impairs lung function or curtails breathing

BENEFITS: Takes over breathing, allowing doctors to concentrate on treating the condition affecting the lungs.

LIMITATIONS: Cannot reverse illness or disease. Simply sustains life.

WHAT HAPPENS IF NOT USED: Breathing slows until it stops. Medication can ease discomfort.

TREATMENT: Tube feeding

PURPOSE: To administer nutrition through a vein or through a tube directly into the stomach

WHEN USED: When an injury or illness prevents swallowing

BENEFITS: Alleviates hunger as well as mental confusion caused by dehydration.

LIMITATIONS: May prolong the dying process for the terminally ill.

WHAT HAPPENS IF NOT USED: Dehydration and starvation. Coma leading to death in one to three weeks.

TREATMENT: Dialysis

PURPOSE: Takes over for the kidneys and removes waste and excess fluid from the body

WHEN USED: During kidney failure

BENEFITS: Prevents waste and excess fluid from damaging other organs.

LIMITATIONS: May require long-term use. Difficult to predict whether kidneys will recover.

WHAT HAPPENS IF NOT USED: Waste buildup in the body eventually leads to coma and heart failure.

In general, there are two reasons to refuse a particular treatment. The first is that the potential benefit of the treatment will not be great enough to justify either its risk or the discomfort that accompanies it. This is the basis for most treatment decisions, and it involves the attitudes that each person brings to the decision. Some people will endure unpleasant and risky treatments for a chance to live longer. Others will trade a longer life for one that's more comfortable, and will allow minimal medical intervention to extend it.

The second reason to refuse medical treatment is the conviction that it will prolong life under intolerable conditions. Even a treatment that causes minimal discomfort might be resisted if it serves only to prolong life in unwanted circumstances. Although a feeding tube may be simple, safe, comfortable, and highly effective in preventing death from starvation and dehydration, some may not want it used if another irreversible condition exists—for example, total body paralysis. Looking at treatments in this light can result in totally different decisions. A treatment that easily passes the risk-benefit or discomfort-benefit test may still be rejected if it serves only to prolong a life that is miserable and without any prospect for improvement.

Most treatment decisions fit easily into one framework or the other, but many decisions are difficult to categorize. Antibiotics for pneumonia are an example. Depending on the circumstances, treatment might involve inserting tubes into the neck or chest to deliver the drug, with only a fair chance of success. Or the antibiotics might come in an easily swallowed pill with a high likelihood of success. Burden-benefit decision making could lead to different choices in these cases.

If some people wish to avoid an uncomfortable treatment that has a low likelihood of fixing a physical problem, others do not want to prolong their lives under certain circumstances. In the latter case, no antibiotic, no matter how simple, would be permitted if the patient had so specified in an accepted living will, since it would probably prolong life. A third possibility complicates the matter: the antibiotic might be viewed as a "comfort measure" since it would ease breathing in an illness that would otherwise cause shortness of breath.

One type of treatment deserves special comment, and not just because it was at the heart of the Terri Schiavo case.

If you are reasonably certain that you would not want intravenous or feeding tubes in certain situations, you should be explicit about those situations. For a person who cannot eat and drink, death is certain unless some means of delivering nutrients and fluids can be put in place. Authorities may differ on whether that kind of death is unpleasant—a coma normally precedes it—but there is unanimity on the final outcome. For this reason, doctors and hospitals are very reluctant to withhold tube feeding because doing so goes against everything they are trained to do, and it might also expose them to a lawsuit. Unless withholding is clearly based on an informed choice made by the patient when she or he had the capacity to decide, the doctor or hospital could respond to the request with defiance or outright refusal.

People see all of these treatment options differently. For some, tube feedings are just another way of ingesting nutrition. What does it matter if food doesn't enter through the mouth as long as it nourishes the body? However, some patient-advocate organizations argue that tube feedings should be subject to the same careful scrutiny as any other medical treatment. It is your business to decide how you feel about tube feedings, and if you want to refuse this treatment under certain circumstances, you should make your views clear in a living will.

For a list of important living will questions, some of them for you and some of them for your lawyer, see the Living Will Legal Consultation quick-reference sheet, reproduced in this chapter and also available as a tear-out sheet at the back of the book. Take it along when you visit your lawyer.

All in the Family

Discussing the terms of a living will with your family is important, even if you meet emotional resistance to the whole idea of talking about death. Despite your best efforts to plan for all eventualities, the actual events might not fit your directives. The best approach in discussing the terms is to be matter-of-fact and reassuring. When you are in crisis and cannot communicate, family members who understand what you want can often help clarify your directives by recollecting specific discussions under specific circumstances. In addition, if you've discussed your wishes with a number of people, those wishes are more likely to be honored.

Reviewing your living will with family members can also help avoid unpleasant scenes and confrontations when you are incapacitated. Even though family members may have little legal authority to make decisions for incapacitated patients, they often feel they have moral authority. They may be confused by statements in a living will that you have not previously shared with them, and they may try to contest your wishes legally if they feel that your choices are not in your best interests.

Having a chat with your family doctor may also be useful before you make decisions about the terms of your living will. Your doctor is likely to be monitoring your hospital care or even caring for you directly

Living Will Legal Consultation
(Make as many photocopies as you need.)

Name of Attorney:

Date and Time of Meeting:

Questions to Resolve before the Meeting

1. Do you want your organs donated?
   Yes   No   Yes, but under the following conditions:

2. If necessary, would you like to be resuscitated?
   Yes   No   Yes, but under the following conditions:

3. Do you want to be kept alive by life support?
   Yes   No   Yes, but under the following conditions:

4. Do you want all pain alleviated, even if it hastens death?
   Yes   No   Yes, but under the following conditions:

5. Would you like to be fed and hydrated through a tube?
   Yes   No   Yes, but under the following conditions:

6. Who will make all your medical decisions if you are unable (medical power of attorney)?
   Name:
   Address:
   Phone Number:

7. Where will copies of the living will be stored (for convenient access)?

Questions for Your Attorney

Are you ethically and morally comfortable preparing a legal document that could end my life?

Can the living will you prepare withstand court challenge in this (state/provincial) jurisdiction or in other jurisdictions outside your own?

Can it be updated easily and inexpensively as needs and preferences change?

Who needs to be notified about the existence of this living will?
    Family:

    Friends:

    Family Physician:

    Clergy:

    Other:

Notes

when your instructions become relevant, and may be predisposed to honor requests communicated directly before you become terminally ill or incapacitated. Your doctor can also help you phrase your requests in a way that makes sense to other doctors and help answer questions you may have about the clinical implications of your requests. Ask your doctor to point out any illogical or inconsistent features in the draft of the living will. Sometimes refusing one kind of treatment makes it unreasonable to expect to receive another kind of treatment—such as antibiotics if you have stipulated no heroic measures in the event of heart failure. Your doctor can also help you create consistent and coherent directives. And make sure your doctor discloses any aspects of your living will that cause him or her discomfort because of personal, moral, or professional constraints. The time to come to an understanding is now, not later.

SMART MOVES: **Prepare a Living Will**

- Discuss the terms of the living will with each member of the family and explain its conditions, being as clear as you can but staying open to questions about your motives for each request so that everyone understands what you want and why you want it.
- Ask your lawyer to help you prepare a document that has the best possible chance of being honored anywhere in the United States and Canada in case an accident or serious illness occurs while you are traveling.
- Make sure everyone in the family knows when a final version has been prepared and signed—and exactly where copies are located.
- Avoid storing copies in locations that cannot be accessed in a hurry, like a bank's safety deposit box, because crises do not follow a nine-to-five schedule.
- Plan to review the living will at least twice a year. Revise and update it as your circumstances and your wishes change.
- Be aware you can change any of its provisions any time. Make sure everyone has up-to-date copies.

- Give your family doctor a copy, and carry a card or note that informs hospital staff that a living will exists.

Assess your loved ones with your living will in mind. As much as you love them, are you confident that all of them will go along with your expressed wishes if they ever have to make tough decisions that might result in your death? Will they waver when they are in danger of losing you? Could your treatment options cause dissension within the family and at the hospital? Doctors and nurses say that conflict often occurs when adult children arrive from out of town feeling guilty that they haven't spent more time with a terminally ill parent. They are resistant to taking steps to end the parent's life, even though a brother or sister who lives nearby says that is what the parent wanted.

If you have any doubts about family members, consider entrusting someone completely outside the family with the right to make decisions on your behalf, someone you're comfortable with. The formal term is *medical power of attorney* (POA), sometimes called *durable power of attorney* or *proxy*. Don't be motivated in your choice by feelings of guilt or obligation. Pick someone who is levelheaded, mature, and calm in a crisis. Selecting someone who lives in the same city that you do could also be helpful. Plan to spend significant time with that person, thoroughly acquainting them with your wishes but also sharing your values and your medical philosophy. Your living will should codify everything you want done or not done, making it an easy reference for the person you've appointed, but you also need to give context—the reasons underlying the decisions reflected by your living will.

Power-of-attorney forms, available from most hospitals. are straightforward. Although you can also integrate your power-of-attorney choice into your living will, even the best living will cannot cover all possible circumstances, so you have to trust your chosen proxy to know you well enough to make the same decisions you would if you were able to. Be sure to let your family and friends know who you chose.

If you don't want to wade into the complications and make the decisions required for a comprehensive living will, you might want to issue a simple do-not-resuscitate order, a form of advance directive that has been around since the 1960s. Health-care professionals, clergy, and lawyers widely accept DNR orders as medically and ethically appropriate. The orders hinge on the right of all patients to make decisions in their own best interests—and those interests may include the desire to avoid emergency efforts to save their lives. Some patients do not want CPR.

Putting on the Brakes

Cardiopulmonary resuscitation—the term is often abbreviated to *resus* (pronounced "resus") by hospital insiders instead of the well-known CPR—refers to the medical procedures used to restart a patient's heart and breathing. These can include basic moves like mouth-to-mouth resuscitation and chest compression using the hands to press the sternum (breastbone) to try to get the heart working again. Advanced CPR may involve using defibrillator paddles to deliver electric shocks to the heart, inserting a tube to open the patient's airway, or injecting quick-start drugs directly into the heart. In extreme cases, the chest can be opened and the heart massaged.

In an emergency, medical professionals assume that the patient would consent to CPR given the choice, and unless they consider CPR futile after making a quick assessment, CPR usually is automatically applied. A do-not-resuscitate (DNR) order tells medical professionals not to perform any form of CPR under any circumstances. Hospital DNR orders instruct medical staff not to revive the patient if the heartbeat and breathing stop. If the patient is in a nursing home or at home, a DNR order tells the staff or emergency medical personnel not to perform resuscitation and not to transfer the patient to a hospital for CPR. While there may be slight variations in language, all DNR orders express the same purpose, and they travel with patients, no matter where they're being treated.

When CPR is successful, it restores the heartbeat and breathing and brings patients back to the same condition they were in before the crisis. It will not cure the cause of the crisis and even if successful could result in lingering side effects. A lot depends on the patient's overall medical condition. Age alone does not determine whether CPR will be successful, although the illnesses and frailties that often accompany aging can reduce the odds. When patients are seriously or terminally ill, CPR may not work either, or it may only partially work, leaving the patient brain-damaged or in worse shape than before the heart stopped. Such patients may refuse aggressive efforts at resuscitation when their hearts stop.

But you may be in reasonable overall health and still want to avoid the possible trauma of resuscitation. You do not have suicidal thoughts, but you may have lived a long and full life by your standards. You may be completely alone in the world and feel ready to go. Or you don't believe that extraordinary efforts to save you would return the kind of benefit that would give you a life worth living by your standards. Whatever your reasons, you are in charge. Anyone legally considered an adult can issue a DNR order—or appoint someone in the family or a proxy to issue it on his or her behalf. Be aware that a DNR order is a decision only about CPR. It does not relate to any other treatment.

There could be a catch. If you are already a hospital patient, some jurisdictions may require the approval of a doctor before your DNR order is formally entered into your chart. That said, you should have a discussion in advance with your family doctor anyway because he or she can confirm that you were of sound mind when you issued the order. You could also incorporate a DNR order into your living will, which might give the order additional weight if challenged. You may want your lawyer to check local laws that could have an impact on your decision.

If you request a DNR order while you are in the hospital, most jurisdictions say that your hospital doctor must follow your wishes or else transfer your care to another doctor who will comply. Typically, any dispute has to be resolved within seventy-two hours, after which the doctor must either enter the order into your chart or transfer care to another doctor. You can also ask for a DNR order to be removed from your chart at any time. That part is easy. You only have to notify your doctor or nurse. You do not even have to do it in writing.

In many jurisdictions, your DNR order will follow you out of the hospital and back to your home. But not in every case. Do not assume that all paramedics will respect your order in all jurisdictions if someone panics and calls an ambulance when you collapse. In some cases, paramedics work for private companies providing a service to the local health authority, and they may not respect a DNR order if it could expose them to a potential lawsuit. Again, consult a lawyer. It may be possible to introduce a clause in your DNR order that releases paramedics from liability. In that case, they might comply with your wishes and make no effort to revive you. They might not even take you to the hospital.

Scary thoughts? Yes. But as you ponder and organize the conditions in a living will or a DNR order, realize that you will be sparing the people you love from having to make decisions at a time when they could be overwhelmed by shock and grief. You may not even be aware of what is happening to you in a medical crisis, but they will. For them to recognize your enormous gift to them may take a while, and their gratitude may be slow in coming, no matter what the outcome. By taking charge of your own life, even if that means possibly shortening it because you choose to, be confident you're acting in your own best interests as well as the best interests of those you love.

4
Surgery
Cutting Through the Confusion

Suppose the surgeon says: "The X-ray shows an unusual mass in your stomach. Although I don't believe it's cancer, given the location and your blood results, I think it would be wise to schedule some exploratory surgery to confirm. It could be a hepatic artery aneurysm or aberrant pancreatic tissue that's been causing you discomfort, but even if the mass turns out to be malignant, I believe we can operate successfully. I don't want to take any risks, though. I think we should schedule the surgery right away. Are you okay with that?"

Here's what the patient might hear: "Bjgjjjth auuuhne mass ggwhh cnncht stomach mammw ahght amm cancer shhnnt ht mbmmghht ksgxn surgery aggdffce dfg malignant dqyycgh jhgh tyuwq risks ghhhjejnymcjjs surgery right away. Are you okay with that?"

It has been estimated that patients facing surgery understand less than half of what doctors tell them. No wonder. They could be frightened and overwhelmed to hear that they might have a serious or lifethreatening condition. The news may be too complicated to understand, even though the procedure could be fairly routine, like a hip replacement. The surgeon may seem to lack the time and forbearance to explain thoroughly.

As you and your loved one navigate through the surgical landscape, you may hear many terms that you don't understand. Don't hesitate to ask for clarification. The glossaries at the back of the book are handy for quick reference and include many specific terms that might come up, as well as many of the terms discussed in this chapter. Here's a helpful hint: *ectomy* at the end of a word means "surgical removal," and *scopy* means "viewing; observing." You will pick up other terms as you talk with the surgeon and other hospital professionals.

The Surgical Consultation

Most busy surgeons exude supreme confidence, a desirable but potentially intimidating quality in someone who wields a very sharp instrument. However, that attitude can sometimes be taken as brusqueness or even arrogance when there's discussion about using that scalpel on someone who could be the most important person in your life. If you are with your nervous loved one when a surgeon is proposing surgery, you can be helpful. You can ask the important questions, press politely but insistently for answers, and record the answers. Start with the following ten questions.

1. What will be done during surgery, and why is it recommended?

Ask for a clear description of the operation and its purpose. Don't be afraid to ask the surgeon to draw a picture to show exactly what the surgery involves. Find out if other surgical procedures might be less invasive. In fact, are there alternatives to surgery? Could medication be an alternative to surgery? Could a change in lifestyle? Sometimes surgery is the only way to fix a problem, but even then, one option might be watchful waiting, to see whether the problem gets better or worse. What will happen if your loved one doesn't have the surgery—will the condition worsen, or could it go away by itself?

2. How will surgery help?

With successful knee or hip replacement your loved one will probably be able to walk comfortably again—and in a reasonably short time. The results of that type of surgery are fairly easy to predict because it is done so frequently and the statistical evidence is encouraging. But the potential benefits of other kinds of surgery might be harder to predict. Still, encourage the surgeon to make a best guess. To what extent will the surgery improve your loved one's health or comfort, and how long will the benefits last? Will the benefits last a lifetime, or will another operation be needed later on? You will want straight answers so that you can have realistic expectations.

3. What are the risks?

All operations carry some risks, and surgeons are required to disclose them fully. The surgeon may rattle through them quickly, but you and your loved one have the right to know exactly what they are, clearly and concisely explained—even down to the known percentage of occurrences of this or that outcome. You both need to weigh the potential benefits against the risks. Ask about the side effects of the operation, too, such as the degree of pain that might be expected and how long that pain will last. Most surgeons tend to soft-pedal the discomfort that can follow some operations—"You'll be back on your feet in no time." But tolerance of pain can vary from person to person, so you should ask for a worst-case scenario.

4. What kind of experience has the surgeon had with this surgery?

How many times has the doctor performed this surgery, and what percentage of the doctor's own patients demonstrated successful results? Surgery is one of those skills for which repetition increases the odds of success. The more experience with a particular surgery, the better. At the Shouldice Hospital in Ontario, for example, all the surgeons do is repair hernias; the procedure has been their single specialty for more than sixty years, and the success rate is measurably very high. To reduce your loved one's risks, you want a doctor who is thoroughly trained in the surgery being proposed and who has plenty of experience doing it.

5. Where will the surgery be done?

Many surgeries today are done on an outpatient basis. Patients go to a hospital or a clinic for the surgery and return home the same day. Other patients require an extended hospital stay because the operation is more complicated. Depending on the surgeon's affiliation, the hospital could be on the other side of town or a long drive from your home and your busy life. You need to know about commuting time if you are going to remain close to your loved one through the process.

6. Will your loved one be put to sleep for the surgery?

The surgery may require only a local or a regional anesthetic—in which case, just part of the body is numbed for a short time, and the patient remains conscious. A general anesthetic puts the patient to sleep. The surgeon should tell you whether a local (just the surgical site itself), regional (a larger area around the site), or general (the entire body) anesthetic will be administered and why this type of anesthesia is recommended for this particular procedure. But the final call rests with the anesthetist, who will meet you and your loved one in a preoperative assessment, which is normally scheduled before any but very minor surgery.

7. How long will the surgery take?

A lot of surgeries can be done with reasonable speed and don't require a prolonged stay in a hospital. Generally speaking, the quicker the surgery, the quicker the recovery. A rule of thumb is that surgeries taking longer than about an hour almost always require a general anesthetic—and since patients need time to recover from the anesthetic itself as well as the surgery, an extended stay may be indicated. Your loved one's surgery may be different, however, so ask. Also ask whether your loved one will need to stay overnight in the hospital—or longer.

8. How long will recovery take, and what can your loved one expect?

You will want to know when most people are able to resume their normal activities after the kind of surgery your loved one is facing. When can your loved one expect to do some simple chores around house? How about returning to work? Just lifting a bag of groceries could stress an incision and cause a setback. The surgeon might hedge on the answer to this question because much will depend on how the surgery goes and how quickly your loved one responds. Ask your surgeon what to expect in the first few days after surgery, as well as in the weeks and months that follow. How long will your loved one be confined to bed, what limitations will be placed on him or her, and what supplies or equipment, if any, will be needed after discharge? Knowing ahead of time what to expect will help you both cope better and will lead to a faster recovery.

9. What will the surgery cost?

Most medically recommended surgeries in Canada are covered by national health insurance, as are many elective surgeries. If you live in the United States, health insurance coverage varies. You may not have to pay anything. You might have a deductible to meet. Or you may have to pay a percentage of the cost. The surgeon's office assistant can usually give you the information you need, but you should also check with your insurance company. Be aware there could be both a surgeon's fee and a hospital or facility fee—you need to know the cost of both. Find out from your insurance company if you are responsible for a flat co-pay—a set amount for the surgery—or if you have to pay a percentage of the bill. There can be a big difference in cost.

10. Should we get a second opinion?

If you have asked all these questions and are not satisfied with the answers or if you are still uncomfortable about proceeding with the surgery, consider seeking a second opinion. Be wary if this surgeon discourages getting a second opinion or suggests that getting one would be a waste of time. A second opinion can be a good way for you to gain perspective on your loved one's surgical options. In fact, many health plans require it—but find out if the cost of a second opinion is covered. If you want a second opinion, find someone who has experience doing that particular surgery; your family doctor may be able to help with a recommendation. But keep in mind that a second opinion will not necessarily be any more enlightening than the first one. And if the two opinions disagree, you and your loved one will still have to weigh the options and pick the one you both feel most comfortable with.

These questions are incorporated in the Surgical Consultation quick-reference sheet (see it nearby in this chapter or at the back of the

Surgical Consultation
(Make as many photocopies as you need.)

Name of Patient and Relationship:

Date and Time of Meeting:

Place of Meeting:

Reason for Proposed Surgery:

Name of Surgeon:

Specialty:

Experience:

Recommended Procedure:

Open Surgery?
    Risks:
    Benefits:

Minimally Invasive (Laparoscopic) Surgery?
    Risks:
    Benefits:

Review of Patient's Medical Records:

Examination of Patient:

Day Surgery:
    Estimated Length of Surgery:
    Estimated Time to Full Recovery:

In-Hospital Surgery:
  Estimated Length of Surgery:
  Estimated Length of Stay:
  Estimated Time to Full Recovery:

Anesthetic Required
  Local:
  Regional:
  General:

Predicted Level of Postoperative Discomfort:
  Mild:
  Moderate:
  Significant:

Scheduled Date and Time of Preoperative Assessment:
  Place of Assessment:

Scheduled Date and Time of Surgery:
  Place of Surgery:

Bring:
  Proof of insurance or health card
  Name of referring physician and contact information
  List of patient's current medications (including herbal remedies and alternative therapies)
  List of patient's known allergies

Notes

book). You may want to fill it in at the appointment and use it as a record of your conversation with the surgeon.

SMART MOVES: **Talking with the Surgeon**

- If working with a pad and pen could be a hassle, bring along a voice recorder and ask the surgeon's permission to use it to record everything that is said.
- Don't monopolize the conversation. You are there to gather information. Encourage your loved one to ask questions and express any additional concerns.
- Ask the surgeon to point you to resources like books and Web sites that might help you understand the procedure being proposed.

It is important to have confidence in the doctor performing the surgery. Whether the surgeon is someone you and your loved one chose or someone you were referred to, take some steps to make sure that he or she is qualified to perform this particular operation. Ask your primary-care doctor, your local medical society, or your health insurance company about the surgeon's experience with the procedure. Ask about the surgeon's credentials: Does the surgeon have certifications that make him or her especially recommended to perform the procedure? Make certain the surgeon is affiliated with an accredited healthcare facility. Where the surgery is being performed is often as important as the person holding the scalpel. Ideally, you want the best possible surgeon operating in a setting with a first-class clinical reputation.

Consider signing a consent form now. Your loved one may then have time to donate blood that could be used during the surgery—and it can be frozen if there is a change in the schedule. Also encourage your loved one to give some thought to creating a living will to reflect his or her wishes about hospital care (see chapter 3).

What Is Surgery?

The American Medical Association defines *surgery* as "the treatment of disease, injury, or other disorders by direct physical intervention, usually with instruments." In other words, a surgeon inflicts a strategic wound on the body for a therapeutic purpose. Done skillfully and under tightly controlled conditions, surgery can restore health or well-being, but there is still a wound from which the body needs to recover. Most people don't realize that the incision required for surgery sometimes requires nearly as much recovery time as the condition the surgery is intended to remedy. The operation is a double whammy.

People typically undergo surgery for one of three reasons. Optional or elective surgery is surgery that may not be essential or urgent. An example is having an unsightly but harmless wart removed. Required surgery corrects a condition that may not be urgent but that is getting in the way of comfortable daily living. An example is removal of painful kidney stones that have resisted medication and other treatments. Emergency surgery is performed when the medical condition is urgent and potentially life-threatening. An example is surgery in a case of acute appendicitis.

More than fifty million North Americans will undergo surgery of some kind in a given year, from the removal of a small facial mole for cosmetic reasons to a life-saving kidney transplant. Surgery can be used to confirm a diagnosis, to take cells or a slice of tissue from a suspicious lump for examination (a biopsy), or to remove diseased tissues or organs in part (a resection) or totally. It can also be used to relieve pain, to implant such mechanical or electronic devices as artificial knees and heart pacemakers, and to repair parts of the body damaged by disease or injury.

Surgical methods have come a long way in the past 50 years. Most surgeries used to involve large incisions because the surgeon needed a full view of the organs or structures being operated on. Open surgeries are still necessary for the removal of major organs and for heart-transplant and heart-bypass operations.

But now the trend is toward minimally invasive surgery, done without a large incision. The benefit? Patients recover faster, with less pain, less blood—and less trauma to the body. That is another reason why you and your loved one should be clear about the surgical options. In the twenty-first century, there is no reason for surgery to hurt more than it has to.

In laparoscopic surgery (sometimes called keyhole or pinhole surgery), operations are performed through very small incisions. The surgeon is guided by a laparoscope, a telescopic rod and lens system, usually connected to a video camera and a television screen, with a fiber optic cable system and a light attached so the surgeon can see inside the body. For abdominal or pelvic operations, the whole area is inflated with carbon dioxide to create a viewing and working field. Various medical tests—any procedure with *scopy* in its name (colonoscopy, trachoscopy, etc.)—use laparoscopic technology.

The technique isn't brand-new. Doctors began experimenting with laparoscopic surgery as early as 1902. Digital camera technology gave it a major boost in the late 1980s. Today surgeries to treat conditions like colon cancer, inflammatory bowel disease, hernias, and brain tumors can be performed without major cuts. And sometimes the surgeon's assistant will be a robot.

First-generation surgical robots are showing up in operating rooms around the world. They are not independent—they still require a human surgeon to manage them by remote control or voice activation—but they integrate with minimally invasive surgical techniques to allow for incredibly precise and tiny movements. So far they have been used to position the lens on the end of a laparoscope, perform gallbladder surgery, and correct conditions like chronic heartburn. They have also been used in certain kinds of heart surgery, where surgeons risk exhaustion and possible hand tremors after long hours at the operating table. Robots don't tire; even the steadiest hand is no match for them.

Surgical robots are amazing to watch, but they have their limits. The technology is still in its infant stage. Because robots respond to human commands, there is often a slight delay before they comply. In most surgeries, that may not be critical, but there is pressure on the robotics industry to develop machines that can virtually erase the pause between command and function.

ASKED AND ANSWERED: The first surgery performed entirely by a robot occurred in Italy in 2006. Robotic surgery is being touted for its potential value in rural areas and nonindustrialized nations, where surgeons in a central hospital could control remote machines in several distant locations.

Two surgical methods that don't use knives at all have also been around for a while, and they, too, are being constantly refined. Some day they may partner with robotics to set the standard for most surgeries. These two methods are laser surgery and electrosurgery.

A laser is a device that emits a concentrated beam of light radiation. A laser beam can cauterize a wound, repair damaged tissue, or destroy cells. With a very narrow laser beam a surgeon can cut through tissue without damaging neighboring cells. The laser is used in place of surgical cutting instruments in eye surgery and gynecological procedures; it can remove skin marks and excise small tumors; and it can be used in other surgeries as well.

In electrosurgery the tools of the surgeon are electrical instruments operating on high-frequency electric currents and generating intense heat; they work in the same manner as the coil in a toaster or hair dryer. The technique is often used to remove lesions or minor skin growths, staunch bleeding, or cut tissue.

ASKED AND ANSWERED: Currently, more than 60 percent of elective surgeries are performed on an outpatient basis in the United States. Health experts predict that rate will rise to nearly 75 percent by 2020.

Risks and Complications

Because surgery is much less invasive than it used to be, a lot of procedures can now be done on an outpatient (or ambulatory) basis. A hospital admission used to be automatic. Now many patients are in and out the same day and escape a long hospital stay. Surgical care in the fast lane has the added benefit of reducing emotional and physical stress on the patient.

Generally, outpatient surgery is appropriate for simple procedures that can be done in under an hour, that need only a local anesthetic, and that don't require close monitoring of the patient afterward. Outpatient surgery offers several benefits over the kind of surgery that normally has to be followed by an inpatient hospital stay. Among them are a lower risk of infection after surgery, a shorter recovery period, recovery at home, fewer delays, shorter waiting times, lower costs, and less disruption of the patient's schedule.

But there is a downside to speeding things up. Same-day surgery imposes more responsibility on the patient to complete the necessary preoperative tests, manage pain medications, keep incisions clean, and follow through with postoperative care. Without family support, for instance, a woman who has small children to care for at home may be unwilling or unable to take on the added responsibility of having same-day surgery.

Even if help is at hand and personal schedules are flexible, not everyone can have outpatient surgery. If a large incision has to be made or if the risk of complications is high, same-day surgery may not be an option. People with chronic conditions like diabetes, heart disease, and hypertension (high blood pressure)—anyone at risk of complications potentially requiring hospitalization—might not be eligible. Inpatient surgery allows clinical staff to keep an eye on the patient's recovery and ensures immediate medical attention in the event of a problem like infection or hemorrhage (bleeding).

Because any kind of surgery involves risks and the prospect of complications, you and your loved one need to know what to expect. You know there will be pain, but you may wonder what your loved one's level of discomfort might be. In general, the amount of discomfort following surgery depends on the type of surgery performed. Some typical discomforts include nausea and vomiting resulting from general anesthesia, a sore throat caused by the tube placed in the trachea (windpipe) for breathing during surgery, and soreness and swelling around the incision site once the anesthetic wears off. Patients can also experience restlessness and sleeplessness, thirst, and either constipation or flatulence.

Shock

One of the most common complications following surgery is shock. Hospital staff will be on high alert for any signs of it. Shock results from a dangerous reduction in blood flow throughout the body, caused by a sharp drop in blood pressure, oxygen, or glucose. Treatments include halting any blood loss, maintaining an open airway, keeping the patient flat, reducing heat loss with blankets, supplying oxygen with a ventilator (respirator) and providing medication.

Blood Loss

Rapid blood loss from the surgery site itself can lead to shock, and the first remedy may be a blood transfusion—a transfer of blood, perhaps the patient's own blood saved from an earlier donation in case of need—often together with infusions of saline solution and plasma preparation, all to help replace fluids. A saline solution, which contains sodium chloride (salt) and sterile water, is normally used in an intravenous drip for dehydrated patients. Plasma is the watery, straw-colored fluid that carries blood cells as they circulate. An intravenous (IV) drip goes directly into a vein.

Infection

Infection, which occurs when bacteria invade the surgical site, is another threat. Infection can spread to adjacent organs and tissue and spread more widely from there, even traveling through the bloodstream to involve the whole body. Infections can delay healing. But antibiotics can usually deal with the problem, and any abscesses—places where pus collects—will be drained as part of cleansing the wound.

ASKED AND ANSWERED: According to a 2005 article in the *Journal of Infectious Diseases,* the risk of surgery-site infection increases steadily from age seventeen to age sixty-five, peaking between sixty-five and seventy-four, and then drops off year by year thereafter. Infection is extremely rare among the very elderly (aged ninety-plus).

Blood Clot

Blood can clot within deep-lying veins. That is called deep vein thrombosis. Large blood clots can break free and clog an artery to the heart, leading to heart failure. Treatment, which depends on the location and size of the blood clot, may include anticoagulant medications (to prevent clots from forming) or thrombolytic medications (to dissolve clots).

Pulmonary (Lung) Complications

Pulmonary complications can occur within forty-eight hours of surgery when patients do not breathe deeply. The lungs can also be affected when the patient inhales food, water, blood, or vomit or catches pneumonia. Symptoms may be wheezing, chest pain, fever, and coughing.

Urine Retention

Temporary urine retention, or the inability to empty the bladder, may also occur after surgery. It is caused by the anesthetic and is usually treated by the insertion of a catheter, a flexible tube, to drain the bladder until the patient regains bladder control.

The Surgical Process

Whether outpatient or inpatient, the surgical process has four formal phases.

1. The *surgical diagnosis* is made after medical tests and evaluations reveal a condition requiring surgery.
2. The *preoperative management phase* lasts from the decision to have surgery to the patient's entry into the operating room. During this second phase a preoperative assessment is made, the patient meets the anesthetist, and the patient also undergoes some basic tests—for example, a test of heart function.
3. The *intraoperative care phase* lasts as long as the patient is in the operating room.

4. The *postoperative management phase* lasts from the transfer to the recovery room until follow-up clinical evaluation, which may occur weeks after the surgery.

Normally, anyone about to undergo very minor outpatient surgery does not have to do much by way of preparation. You and your loved one just have to show up for the appointment. You are there to give moral support—and to drive the patient home afterward. That is important because any kind of surgery is stressful, and your loved one could be disoriented by the experience. Bring a favorite book to read while you wait. It will help relieve boredom and anxiety.

If your loved one is scheduled for more serious surgery, and especially if a general anesthetic is indicated, you can lend support by keeping a record of visits and organizing the various blood tests, X-rays, electrocardiograms, and any other procedures that have to take place prior to surgery. The surgeon's office will provide a complete list and help you book appointments. The Preoperative Assessment quick-reference sheet (reproduced nearby and at the back of the book) will help you keep track for either outpatient or inpatient surgery.

What to Take and Avoid before the Operation

If your loved one is a smoker and will be having general anesthesia, he or she will be advised to stop smoking as far in advance of surgery as possible. Because vomiting during the procedure could be dangerous, it is likely that no food or drink will be allowed after midnight the day before surgery; if the operation is scheduled for Thursday, that means no food or drink after midnight on Wednesday, but sipping a small amount of water could be okay—check with a nurse in the surgery unit. Depending on the kind of surgery, the surgeon may also want the patient to have an enema the night before the surgery to cleanse the bowels. This isn't a pleasant task, but you can help if you are not squeamish.

In the days leading up to surgery, you can encourage your loved one to eat a well-balanced diet including plenty of foods rich in vitamin C, which may help promote tissue healing. Regular exercise will help build energy and maintain strength. Some experts also recommend

Preoperative Assessment
(Make as many photocopies as you need.)

Location of Assessment Clinic:
    Phone Number:

Date and Time of Appointment:

Nurse in Charge of Assessment:

Blood Tests Required?
    Results:

Blood Pressure Reading Required?
    Results:

EKG Required?
    Results:

X-Rays Required?
    Results:

Results of Anesthetic Consultation:

Type of Anesthetic Proposed: Local   Regional   General

Scheduled Date, Time, and Place of Surgery:

Scheduled Date, Time, and Place of Follow-up with Surgeon:

Remember:
No food or drink (except water) after midnight before surgery
No alcohol 24 hours before surgery

Bring:

Proof of insurance

Name of family doctor and contact information

List of patient's current medications (including herbal remedies and alternative therapies)

List of patient's known medication allergies

Surgeon's notes and assessment requisition (if given to the patient to take to the assessment)

Notes

avoiding aspirin or aspirin-like medications for seven days prior to surgery because they can interfere with blood clotting. See the Pre-surgery Medications Checklist quick-reference sheet for a list of medications you can take and should not take. (It is reproduced nearby, but you might want to tear out the duplicate checklist at the back and put it on your refrigerator or bulletin board.) Ask your doctor first, though; medical advice personalized for your loved one preempts anything you might read in this book.

Operation Day

The day of surgery has arrived. At the hospital, you and your loved one will meet with the medical team involved in the surgery, including the surgeon, the anesthetist, and other health-care professionals. There may be a brief physical exam. At this point, your loved one could be asked to sign a consent form if that hasn't been done yet.

SMART MOVES: **Getting Ready for the Surgery**

- Bathe or clean the area to be operated on.
- Remove makeup, nail polish, and contact lenses.
- Leave valuables and jewelry at home.
- Bring all appropriate insurance information.
- Bring your loved one's living will or related documents.
- Carry loose, comfortable clothes for your loved one to wear after surgery.
- Advise the medical staff of dentures or other prosthetic devices your loved one may be wearing.

Before entering the operating room, your loved one can expect to change into a hospital gown, receive an identification bracelet, and have an IV line inserted into the forearm for anesthetics and other medications. Then comes transportation on a gurney to the operating room. You will not be allowed any farther than the doors leading to the surgical area. That is when you have to step back and wait—the hard part.

Presurgery Medications Checklist
(Make as many photocopies as you need.)

Prior to Surgery, Patients Can Take:
    Heart medications
    Antireflux medications (Prilosec, Nexium, Protonix)
    Seizure medications (anticonvulsants)
    Anti-hypertensives (blood pressure medications)
    Bronchodilators (inhalers and medications for the lungs)
    Birth control pills
    Steroids (prednisone)
    Immunosuppressants
    Thyroid replacement (Synthroid)
    Anti-Parkinson medications
    COX-2 antagonists (Vioxx, Celebrex)
    Opiates (without aspirin; Tylenol #3, Vicodin, fentanyl, etc.)

Prior to Surgery, Patients *Should Not* Take:
    Chewable antacids (Tums, Rolaids, etc.)
    Diuretics (water pills, furosemide, hydrochlorothiazide)
    Insulin
    Oral hypoglycemics (Glucophage, Avandia, Actos, DiaBeta,
        Micronase, Glucotrol, Amaryl)
    Aspirin (and compounds that contain ASA)
    Nonsteroidal anti-inflammatory drugs (ibuprofen, Motrin, Advil,
        Mobic, Orudis, etc.)
    Potassium
    Weight reduction agents
    Vitamins
    Herbal supplements

Notes

ASKED AND ANSWERED: The value of praying for a patient's recovery has long been a subject of various studies, often with contradictory results. The largest study so far was undertaken in 2006 by scientists at Harvard Medical School. It followed 1,800 heart-surgery patients at six medical centers and concluded that prayer made no apparent difference to outcomes—and that many patients actually suffered increased complications when they knew they were being prayed for.

Your loved one will be looking around at an unfamiliar room before the anesthetic is administered. All the intimidating equipment has a purpose.

- The operating table in the center of the room can be raised, lowered, and tilted in any direction.

- The operating lamp above it allows for brilliant illumination without shadows during surgery.

- Various monitors keep track of heart rate, blood pressure, and other vital measurements. Some of the monitors may be attached to the patient.

- A breathing machine, or ventilator, stands at the head of the operating table. It will give your loved one full oxygen support during the surgery.

- Sterile instruments to be used during surgery are arranged on a stainless steel table.

- A diathermy machine to control bleeding is usually present.

- A heart-lung machine or other specialized equipment may also be in the operating room.

Other items, some not readily apparent, may be available to patients during or after surgery. They represent new advances in medical technology.

BISPECTRAL INDEX (BIS) MONITOR: A device that analyzes the patient's brain wave pattern and converts it into a "depth of sedation" number so the anesthetist can continuously monitor brain function during the operation.

SCOPOLAMINE PATCH: A prescription drug that helps prevent nausea and vomiting associated with motion sickness. The patch is now being used to prevent nausea and vomiting during or after major (inpatient) surgery and is considered useful in preventing aspiration (the inhalation of gastric contents into the lungs and the lower airways). If your loved one has been admitted to the hospital, the small patch would be placed behind the ear the night before surgery, allowing medication to be absorbed through the skin and travel directly into the bloodstream.

REMIFENTANIL: A pain reliever for inducing and maintaining general anesthesia during surgery. The drug breaks down in the bloodstream and body tissues very quickly and safely. Because enzymes break down remifentanil in the blood and muscles, rather than in the liver and kidneys, like other drugs, patients wake sooner, and breathing tubes can be removed sooner.

FIBRIN SEALANTS: A new class of sealants, made from plasma, that help to stop oozing from small blood vessels during surgery when conventional surgical techniques are not feasible. The sealants, which form a flexible shield over the oozing blood vessel, help control bleeding within minutes.

Once the operation is completed and staff are satisfied that the patient is stable, your loved one will be taken to the surgical recovery room, sometimes called the post-anesthesia care unit (PACU). That is where you can join your loved one again and perhaps be the first familiar face she or he sees. You can start by offering reassurance and encouragement. Hold your loved one's hand. Stroke the forehead.

Clinical staff will closely observe their patient's gradual revival from anesthesia. How long revival takes depends on the type of surgery performed and the individual patient's response to it and to the various medications. The clinical staff will:

monitor vital signs, such as blood pressure, pulse, and breathing
look for signs of complications
take the patient's temperature
check for gagging or vomiting
monitor the patient's level of consciousness
check any lines, tubes, or drains
check the wound
check intravenous infusions
monitor the patient's urinary evacuation
maintain the patient's comfort with pain medication and body po-
     sitioning

You can help your loved one's progress by offering to join the staff's efforts to encourage certain breathing and moving exercises in the recovery room. The staff will probably not ask you themselves. They may not want to impose a burden on a family member, or they may think you will get in the way, but many will welcome your offer and open the circle of care around your loved one. They know the clinical side of things. You know the patient—when to nudge and when to pull back. That can be useful in the critical early hours after surgery.

Lying flat for an extended period of time can cause fluids to accumulate in the lungs—and post-surgical patients are particularly vulnerable. Taking deep breaths that use the entire diaphragm and abdomen can prevent pneumonia from setting in. Mild and controlled coughing helps too, because it encourages the removal of fluids from the lungs.

Changing the patient's position helps stimulate circulation by promoting deep breathing and relieving areas under pressure. Moving the legs and feet also stimulates circulation. Your loved one might be encouraged to bend the knees and raise each foot several times, mimicking the motion of pedaling a bike, or to draw circles in the air with the big toe.

Chances are, your loved one will not want to cooperate with any part of this. After surgery, most patients are groggy and confused or cranky. They want everyone to go away so they can go back to sleep and pretend the surgery never happened. But you are there to help them return from a strange and traumatic place. And when you get that first tentative smile, you will know you are exactly where you belong.

5
Intensive Care
Life on the Edge

Florence Nightingale was superintendent of nursing for British military hospitals during the Crimean War in the mid-1850s. Shortly after her appointment, she announced that it was time to introduce a new level of care. She believed that soldiers recovering from major surgery or serious illness would do much better if they were closely attended by nurses in an area apart from other hospital patients, where they would be protected from infection—common among hospitalized battlefield casualties. And because their conditions could change rapidly, she reasoned that they would benefit if they were constantly watched. She called this special area a monitoring unit. When senior medical personnel gave reluctant approval to test the idea, she proved skeptics wrong: hospital mortality rates dropped from 40 percent to 2 percent over the course of the war.

Not until a hundred years later did her groundbreaking idea take hold in North American hospitals. The continent's first intensive-care unit (ICU) opened at the Dartmouth-Hitchcock Medical Center in New Hampshire in 1955. Now most hospitals of any size have at least one.

The staff in modern ICUs may have a lot more medical knowledge and technology at their command than Nightingale did, but they haven't strayed from her original vision. Their first priority is to prolong life. They exist to deliver the highest possible level of care to the

sickest of patients, and they usually do that in an environment that's isolated from the rest of the hospital. The attention provided is very personal, with an average of no more than two patients per nurse. Compare
that to the ten-to-one ratio typical in hospital recovery wards.

Although small hospitals and rural hospitals may not have an ICU,
large community and university-based medical centers may have several—specializing in trauma, cardiovascular, respiratory, surgical, or
neurological patients. Critically ill children are not normally admitted
to an adult ICU. Instead, they're transferred to a local medical center
with a pediatric ICU or to a children's hospital.

> **ASKED AND ANSWERED:** Canada has approximately 6.7 ICU
> beds per 100,000 people. The United States has nearly four
> times as many—25 beds per 100,000 people.

Most modern ICUs have roughly the same layout, with a limited
number of beds, most of them easily visible from a central nursing station. In some hospitals, the ICU is strategically located a short distance
from both the emergency department and the operating rooms of the
surgical department. Visitor access is often restricted, and some ICUs
even keep their doors locked against the possibility of noisy, germ-car-
rying intruders. Sometimes a wall phone hangs beside the ICU entrance with a notice alongside requiring visitors to identify themselves
before they are allowed in.

Why Patients End Up in an ICU

After something like an organ transplant or complex heart surgery your
loved one may need to spend time in an ICU for follow-up care. But
there are other reasons for an ICU stay, all of them potentially life-
threatening. Among the most typical are the following.

Shock

Shock occurs when there is a sudden and severe drop in oxygen, blood pressure, or glucose, resulting in the inability of body organs to function normally. Shock has many causes. Here are the four most common causes and their treatments:

HYPOVOLEMIC SHOCK: Results from severe dehydration or massive blood loss. Treatment: intravenous fluids (IV) and/or blood transfusions.

CARDIOGENIC SHOCK: Results when a weakened heart is not pumping enough blood to meet the body's needs. Treatment: medications or devices to improve heart function

SEPTIC SHOCK: Results when a severe infection causes organ failure. Treatment: intravenous fluids and medications to increase blood pressure and treat the infection

SYSTEMIC INFLAMMATORY RESPONSE SYNDROME (SIRS): Results from massive trauma to the body, which can be caused by a car accident or other incident, a severe infection, or a medical condition, such as pancreatitis. Treatment: intravenous fluids and medications to increase blood pressure

If shock cannot be reversed in a matter of days, the body's organs will start to shut down, with death the likely result.

Acute Respiratory Failure

The lungs remove carbon dioxide from the blood and replace it with oxygen, an efficient exchange system that can suddenly stop functioning. Acute respiratory failure may be the reason for admission to an ICU, but it may also be a complication that occurs in the ICU itself. Pneumonia and heart failure, among other conditions, can cause it. Respiratory failure is usually treated with oxygen and respiratory therapy to help strengthen breathing and clear the lungs of phlegm.

Moderate respiratory failure can be caused by severe pneumonia or chronic obstructive pulmonary disease (COPD). Usually patients with moderate respiratory failure need some type of mechanical support to help them breathe. A patient may wear a tight-fitting face mask that delivers oxygen under pressure from a ventilator (respirator) or have an endotracheal tube (a breathing tube connected to a ventilator) inserted into the mouth and down into the trachea (windpipe).

The most severe form of acute respiratory failure is called acute respiratory distress syndrome (ARDS). The lungs of a patient with ARDS can't supply oxygen to the blood, so a ventilator is usually needed. ARDS has a long list of causes. The common ones are pneumonia, aspiration of foreign matter (vomit, food, etc.) into the lungs, trauma, severe infection, and pancreatitis. There is no single therapy for ARDS. The goal is to support the patient until the lungs heal.

Chronic Respiratory Failure

If patients remain critically ill for a long time, they can become very weak and lose the ability to breathe on their own. The respiratory muscles need to be exercised and slowly rebuilt before the patients can breathe on their own again, a process that may take as long as two to three months. When a ventilator is needed for more than a few weeks, it may be necessary to move the tube from the mouth or nose to the neck above the trachea. In that case, a minor surgical procedure called a tracheotomy is performed: a small incision is made in the neck, and the tube is inserted through the incision. This is done to reduce the risk of infection, ease the chance of damage to the trachea from the constant presence of the ventilator tube, improve patient comfort, and help restore lung function. A feeding tube may also need to be inserted.

Sepsis and Severe Sepsis

Major infections are a common cause of ICU admission. Unfortunately, they're also a frequent complication among ICU patients who are already there with other problems.

Sepsis is an extreme infection, and it can develop very quickly. Usually, the body's own defense system fights infection. But in a patient with severe sepsis the body's normal response to infection appears to go berserk, leading to widespread inflammation and blood clotting in tiny vessels throughout the body. Infection often attacks the organs and even the blood. When it invades the bloodstream, it is called septicemia (blood poisoning).

Any kind of infection—bacterial, parasitic, or fungal—anywhere in the body can trigger sepsis. Sepsis can strike anyone at any age, but the very old, the very young, people with preexisting medical conditions, and hospital patients can be particularly vulnerable. It can also result when an immune system has been compromised by chemotherapy or by the drugs used to enable an organ transplant. But it also shows up in patients who have undergone major surgery or suffered any kind of major physical trauma that has affected the body's innate ability to defend itself.

Sepsis and severe sepsis are usually treated with aggressive antibiotics, fluids, and other medications. To keep the body functioning during treatment, the patient often receives ventilation and dialysis (to do some of the work of the lungs and kidneys, respectively).

ASKED AND ANSWERED: The Society of Critical Care Medicine reports that sepsis strikes an estimated 750,000 people every year in the United States alone. As the population ages, that figure is expected to rise to 1,000,000 cases a year by 2015.

Renal (Kidney) Failure

Renal failure is very common in the ICU, and it can also be the reason the patient was admitted to the ICU in the first place. The kidneys normally remove water and toxins from the body, but they often respond to severe illness by shutting down.

Two things happen with renal failure.

First, when the kidneys do not do remove water, extra water accumulates in the body, and it is stored in the skin. The result is swelling of the arms, legs, and face (edema), making the patient look puffy. That extra water also builds up in the organs, impairing their function, and it can even interfere with breathing.

Second, the kidneys no longer remove toxins from the body. The toxins build up, affecting the brain. The patient gets sleepy and often slides into a coma. But these toxins do no lasting harm to the brain, and the patient should regain consciousness when the toxins are removed. Left untreated, the patient may die if the toxins build up enough to stop the heart.

Renal failure is usually rated either mild or severe. Mild cases can be treated with intravenous fluids or medications to help the kidneys work more efficiently. But severe renal failure calls for dialysis, using a machine that takes over the function of the kidneys and removes the toxins and the extra water. Dialysis does not make the kidneys recover faster—the kidneys have to heal by themselves. Dialysis only allows the body to stay alive while the kidneys are improving. Most ICUs have at least one dialysis machine on standby.

There are two types of dialysis: intermittent and continuous. Intermittent dialysis is administered three to four hours a day or every other day. With continuous dialysis the patient is connected all the time. Very ill patients are more likely to need continuous dialysis and will stay hooked up until the kidneys start functioning on their own again.

But will the kidneys completely recover after renal failure? There are obvious variables, but the odds favor patients who had normal kidney function before they got sick. If their kidneys did not function normally before they entered the ICU, the chances of full kidney recovery are worse. It is also true that kidneys can take months to improve; some ICU patients discharged while still on dialysis might continue to need it on an outpatient basis and then recover later.

Neurological Conditions

The staff in ICUs treat a lot of traumatic brain injuries and strokes that can cause behavior changes when a patient is critically ill, but behavior changes can happen from other causes, too. A patient may be sleepy, disoriented, frightened, or agitated whatever the illness. Although some patients may not be awake at all while they remain critically ill, conscious ICU patients flattened by traumatic illness or injury may assume that everything they value has been devastated as well. They imagine that loved ones have died, and the ICU is where they will end their own lives. ICU-induced depression is not rare. When life feels like ground zero in a global disaster, even nurses may be treated with fear and mistrust. Some patients require calming medications and even restraints to prevent self-harm. Patient reactions to being in the ICU will vary depending on the severity of the illness, and any psychological discomfort usually dissipates if the overall condition improves. Elderly patients are extremely susceptible to depression when they find themselves in the unfamiliar environment of an ICU, a condition worsened by the frequent disruption of sleep patterns due to the high level of ambient noise and the brightly lit environment, which appears to have no distinct day or night.

Bleeding and Clotting

Critically ill patients can develop bleeding from the stomach, usually the result of a stress ulcer. Most are given medication to prevent ulcers, but bleeding may occur anyway. The bleeding usually stops by itself, but the patient often requires blood transfusions and sometimes surgery to resolve the problem.

ICU patients are also at risk for developing blood clots in their legs and lungs. Most critically ill patients are given medications or else devices are placed on their legs to prevent clotting, but it can still happen. Minor blood clots can be treated with anticoagulation drugs, but severe cases can be life-threatening.

Multiple Organ Dysfunction Syndrome (MODS)

Any critical illness that brings a patient to the ICU has the potential to affect the other organs in the body—a nasty demonstration of the domino theory. Slowly one organ after another can start to fail, a condition called multiple organ dysfunction syndrome. There is no specific treatment for MODS; the only option is supportive care. Usually the lungs and the kidneys are the first to go, followed by the brain and then the immune system. Other organs and systems get involved at that point—the heart, the liver, the blood, the intestines, and so on. The body shuts down, organ by organ. Once a patient develops MODS, the odds of survival decrease as the organs fail.

ASKED AND ANSWERED: The popular assumption that most ICU patients die is not true. In a 2006 report provided by the U.S. Department of Health and Human Services, the average ICU mortality rate ranges from 12 to 17 percent, depending on a complex mix of variables that includes severity of the illness.

Strange Place, Strange Face

When you visit a loved one in the ICU for the first time, it is natural to feel anxious. You won't know what to expect. You won't know what to say. Nor will your discomfort be eased by what you see and hear as you enter the unit.

Depending on the time of day, you may see a lot of doctors and nurses bustling back and forth, most of them looking surprisingly cheerful despite being in a place where life often hangs in the balance. The mood has a startling buoyancy, and you may even hear the occasional wisecrack between professionals. Don't be fooled. The staff work under extreme pressure and are profoundly committed to delivering extraordinary care. Sometimes they let off steam, but they are never as casual as they might seem.

Where is the sober dimness you expected, and the solemn hush? The light appears to be brighter than anywhere else in the hospital, and all those life-support machines working together provide an overlay of noise. In fact, they produce a decibel level that has been compared to what people hear when they're standing next to a busy highway.

And then there are the chirps and beeps and buzzes.

Patients and families can be worried when alarms go off. Almost every piece of equipment that monitors patient functions has an alarm. The nursing staff select what body functions to monitor and set the limits or parameters for each alarm. Remember that an alarm almost never signals an emergency. Instead, it alerts the staff that the patient needs closer attention or an immediate intervention to prevent an emergency. Alarms are just another set of tools that the staff use to assist in the care of your loved one. If you visit the ICU with any frequency, you will get used to them.

S M A R T   M O V E S : **Your ICU Visit**

- Always wash your hands before entering the ICU. Sinks or disinfectant dispensers are usually located near the entrance to the unit.
- Never bring flowers or food into the ICU. They are considered potential sources of infection. If you bring any, you will have to leave them behind in the waiting room.
- Avoid wearing aftershave or cologne. Some scents, even those normally familiar to the patient, can cause nausea, depending on the extent of the illness and the treatments being used.
- Respect the privacy of other patients by looking straight ahead as you pass by their open cubicles or rooms.
- Identify yourself to the nurses looking after your loved one and tell them a detail or two about the patient that will personalize the nurse-patient relationship.
- Always wash your hands before touching the patient to prevent infection, and ask for a pair of disposable plastic or latex gloves, which are often recommended as an extra precaution. Most ICU rooms or cubicles have a sink nearby, as well as a supply of gloves.

Get ready to be startled when you see your loved one. For a brief moment you may not even recognize the patient you came to visit. That's a normal reaction. Your loved one may look pale and diminished, with no hint of the vibrancy you're used to, and you may find yourself wondering if full recovery is even possible. Other things may puzzle and distress you. Here are some examples of what you might see.

Bruising

Intensive-care patients require a large number of blood tests, many of which are performed daily. Even when the blood for lab tests is drawn correctly, bruising may occur. A lot of critical illnesses make patients prone to bruising because blood clotting is one of the potential side effects. Patients with liver problems, infections, or poor nutrition also bruise easily. The elderly and people who have been on blood thinners are prone to bruising as well. And the face may have bruising and swelling after head or brain surgery.

Swelling

Frequently the inability to move, the assisted breathing, the critical illness, and the treatments for blood pressure may together cause swelling (edema) in the face and body. Sometimes the eyes swell, and the inside lining of the eyelid protrudes with the swelling. Little can be done to prevent all this. The nurses may try to decrease the effect by keeping the head of the bed slightly raised and the hands elevated on pillows. They may remove rings to protect the blood flow to the fingertips.

Oozing

In some critical illnesses, a pale fluid may ooze out of the puncture sites where blood has been drawn and out of any break or tear in the skin. The oozing results from the accumulation of fluid in the tissues. The fluid, usually straw-colored, is plasma, the liquid part of blood, that has leaked or been pushed into the tissues because of bed rest, ventilator breathing, liver failure, heart failure, or poor nutrition.

Skin Tears

Skin tears can occur when bandages and tapes are removed from the skin, even though the nurses will use the gentlest tape or bandage available that will still adhere to the skin. Bandages (called dressings by staff) are obviously necessary over wounds, but they also keep intravenous lines and other tubes in place. Skin tears are often unavoidable in people who have taken steroids, who have a history of smoking, or who have poor nutrition. The frail elderly are also at risk.

Mucus and Blood

At times there could appear to be a lot of mucus and even blood around the insertion points of the tubes. The nurse will gently clean these areas, but some blood may remain. This is not uncommon in the ICU, and there should be less blood and mucus as the patient recovers.

Skin Pockets

Sometimes small pockets are created under the skin to hold internal monitors: permanent pacemakers, automatic defibrillators, or other devices.

Opening in the Abdomen

Occasionally an opening is made in the wall of the abdomen to allow evacuation of urine or feces. This is a urostomy (for urine evacuation) or a colostomy (for bowel evacuation). Each opening may be temporary or permanent, depending on the reason for its presence.

Weights

If the patient has a broken leg or hip, weights may be rigged to keep the bones straight. The traction will prevent the patient from moving without assistance.

Bedsores

Bedsores occur when skin compromised by severe illness remains in contact with a surface (like a bedsheet) for too long. Bedsores are very painful, and they are completely preventable with simple but attentive care. The best ICUs automatically move every patient every two hours. Ask the nurse if your loved one will be routinely moved to help prevent bedsores from developing. The question is important—the answer could make a major difference to your loved one's comfort.

Tubes and Other Attachments

A confusing array of tubes and lines and pads may be connected to your loved one, adding to your bewilderment and distress. They all have a purpose.

ARTERIAL LINE: A small tube inserted into an artery to continuously monitor blood pressure.

BLOOD PRESSURE CUFF: a large cuff placed on the arm or the leg that may be automatically or manually inflated in order to evaluate the amount of pressure in the arteries.

CENTRAL LINE, PULMONARY ARTERY (PA) CATHETER: A catheter in the neck, chest, or groin that helps in monitoring and treating the flow of blood and may be used to deliver nutrition and medications.

CHEST TUBE: A tube inserted between the chest wall and the lungs to remove free air or blood that may make it difficult for the patient to breathe.

DIALYSIS CATHETER: A tubelike catheter inserted into a large vein in the groin or neck and hooked up to external tubing and then to a dialysis machine for kidney support.

ENDOTRACHEAL TUBE (ETT): A breathing tube inserted through the mouth or nose and connected to a ventilator.

FOLEY CATHETER: A thin, sterile tube inserted into the bladder to drain urine into a bag.

HEART MONITOR LEADS: Sticky pads placed on the chest of almost every ICU patient and attached to a machine to monitor the electrical activity of the heart.

INTRA-AORTIC BALLOON PUMP (IABP): A pump connected to a catheter inserted into the groin to help the heart pump blood.

INTRACRANIAL PRESSURE (ICP) CATHETER: A small tube (catheter) inserted into the brain to monitor brain swelling or to drain excess fluid from the brain. The procedure for inserting the tube through the skull is called a ventriculostomy.

NASOGASTRIC (NG) TUBE: A tube inserted through the nose and down into the stomach or intestines to provide nutrition and remove gastric acid or secretions.

PERIPHERAL LINE: A small plastic tube placed into a vein and used to deliver fluid or medications.

PULSE OXIMETER: A small probe attached to the finger, nose, or ear that helps monitor both the oxygen in the blood and the pulse.

TRACHEOSTOMY TUBE: A breathing tube inserted in the neck when ventilator-assisted breathing is needed for a long period of time.

ASKED AND ANSWERED: The average length of stay (LOS) for a patient in an ICU is five to six days, but thirty-day stays are not uncommon, and some patients have remained for more than a year because their conditions were considered too perilous to be treated as chronic and therefore manageable elsewhere in the hospital or at home.

Restraints

If the patient requires a tube inserted into the mouth, the hands may have to be restrained because of the natural impulse to gag and then attempt to pull out the tube. The ICU staff will do all they can to avoid restraining the patient, but keeping the tube in place is vital. The insertion can be unpleasant to watch because there will be natural resistance, and I advise avoiding it.

Unfamiliar Behavior Patterns

When ICU patients regain consciousness, they may feel confused about where they are and why they're there. They may not know what circumstances brought them to the ICU. They could be anxious and in pain. They may fight the ventilator, try to pull out tubes, and push the nurses away. Fear and discomfort are normal ICU responses, and they can be greatly eased with sedatives and pain medications. But you can help too.

Gauge your loved one's responses, including responses to casual comments about the family and the weather and that day's events at home. If you continue to see confusion or lack of awareness, alert the nurses immediately, even if your loved one appears to be fully conscious. The nurses must count on your personal knowledge of the patient to help them determine whether your loved one's uncharacteristic responses are simply a reaction to the drugs or a sign that something more serious is happening. Critical illness and the medications used to treat it cause chemical changes in the body that can result in strange behavior. It may not be strange to the nurses, but if it seems strange to you, speak up.

Your loved one may not talk to you, but don't be alarmed, especially if a breathing tube is present. It passes close to the vocal cords and impedes speech. Sedatives and pain medications may mean that you're trying to converse with a person who is awake but not fully conscious. Does that mean you should stop trying to communicate? Not for a second. Keep your voice calm and reassuring—and know that your loved one has to reach out through a dense fog to connect with you. If the brain has been injured either by stroke or by trauma, the ability to speak or even to stay awake may have been affected. This is common in the first few days, and as much as a week may pass before doctors can determine whether speech recovery is possible.

Keep talking anyway, even when your loved one drifts away, apparently asleep. There is strong evidence to suggest that critically ill patients hear and remember more than we suspect. Strong evidence also suggests that a familiar voice can be therapeutic. You are your loved one's link to the world outside the scary place he or she is in, and the sound of your voice can be comforting.

SMART MOVES: **Dealing with Patient, Nurses, and Family**

- If you run out of things to say, try reading to your loved one in a gentle voice from a favorite book.
- If your loved one is unable to speak, phrase questions so they can be answered with a nod (yes) or a headshake (no), or even with eye blinks.
- Ask the nurses if you can help with basic tasks like grooming and personal care. That way you can reconnect with your loved one in a tangible way.
- Check in by phone with the nursing station every morning. Ask the person on duty to let your loved one's nurse know when you'll be in to visit that day.
- Touch or hold your loved one's hand. Touch can be very reassuring.
- Bring photographs of your family for display near your loved one's bed. They can be comforting for the patient—and they also tell the nurses something about the person with the complex medical condition.
- If you observe any alarming reactions or behavior, notify the nurse immediately—and then stay well out of the way of staff trying to assess and resolve the problem.
- If you're willing and able, appoint yourself the family spokesperson—the one who fields questions about your loved one and interacts with the care team. With family and friends to update, you might find it handy to fill in the Giving Updates to Family and Friends: Contact Information quick-reference sheet at the back of the book and carry it with you (the form is also reproduced nearby).

Giving Updates to Family and Friends: Contact Information
(Make as many photocopies as you need.)

Name:

City/Town:

Relationship to Patient:

Home Number:

Work Number:

Cell Phone Number:

Pager Number:

Good Times to Call:

Notes (health issues, work/stress issues, etc.):

Name:

City/Town:

Relationship to Patient:

Home Number:

Work Number:

Cell Phone Number:

Pager Number:

Good Times to Call:

Notes (health issues, work/stress issues, etc.):

- But also line up a backup person to step in when you need a break. If caregiver help from family and friends is available, list their names and contact information on the Surrogate Caregivers: Who, What, When quick-reference sheet (also reproduced nearby and at the back of the book).

The ICU Care Team—Who Does What

You will have questions and comments. You may think of ways to help make your loved one more comfortable. And since you will want to ask your questions and offer your suggestions, you should get to know the people on the ICU care team.

Intensivists

Intensivists are the doctors in charge of your loved one's ICU care. They're the experts, board-certified in a medical specialty—surgery, internal medicine, pediatrics, or anesthesiology—and with additional training and certification that qualifies them as specialists in critical care. Intensivists are usually assigned to the ICU full-time, and they work with other critical-care team members to provide patients with ongoing and consistent attention. These doctors know how specific treatments affect organ systems in a critically ill patient, and they oversee all ICU procedures and medications. They may also coordinate the administration of the ICU by setting policies and developing protocols that upgrade professional-practice standards in the ICU, and call in specialists for consultation if needed.

Critical-Care Nurses

Critical-care nurses provide a high level of skilled nursing for total patient care, and they often facilitate communication among all of the people involved with the patient, including families. Their continuous presence encourages early recognition of subtle but significant changes in patient condition, and their clinical awareness of the patient could

Surrogate Caregivers: Who, What, When
(Make as many photocopies as you need.)

Name:

Phone Number:

Days and Times Available:

Willing to:
    Feed the Patient:
    Groom the Patient:
    Read to the Patient:
    Supply Music for the Patient:
    Assist in Bedside Tasks (moving the patient, etc.):
    Other:

Patient's Comments:

Staff Comments:

prevent conditions from worsening and minimize the complications that can arise from critical illness or injury. Because of their close contact with the family and the patient, critical-care nurses often serve as the patient's advocate and become integral to the decision making of the patient, family, and critical-care team. They contribute to morning medical rounds—the formal bedside review of each patient's condition, usually led by an intensivist accompanied by other doctors, some of whom may be residents if the hospital is a teaching facility.

Pharmacist or Clinical Pharmacologist

A pharmacist or clinical pharmacologist is a board-certified specialist in the science and clinical use of medications. The pharmacist with specialty training in ICU care is equipped to recognize needs and problems specific to the critical-care patient and works with members of the health-care team to encourage effective and safe medication therapy.

Registered Dietitian

During a critical illness, the body has additional nutritional requirements, and the patient may require tube feeding. The dietitian assists the team in deciding on the best nutritional plan for the patient and is available for ongoing consultations with nurses as well as families. The dietitian is a good person to know if you have concerns about any food allergies your loved one may have or if you have some taste suggestions that might stimulate appetite. The strategy is to use food to support the goal of recovery.

Social Worker

Often taken for granted, a social worker can add significant value to the ICU interdisciplinary team by providing a link between the clinical care of the patient and the social and emotional needs of patients and their families. The best ICU social workers are superb diplomats who can help resolve family disputes and ease the sudden transition from the

ICU to a recovery floor. Social workers can also help families come to terms with an unsettling diagnosis and guide them to additional resources if needed.

Respiratory Therapists

Respiratory therapists work with the ICU team to help get the patient breathing normally again, using oxygen therapy, ventilator management, aerosol medication therapy, cardiorespiratory monitoring, and patient and family education.

Physical Therapist (in Canada: Physiotherapist)

The physical therapist helps restore limb function, improve mobility, relieve pain, and prevent or limit permanent physical disabilities. Keeping ICU patients as mobile as possible is important, down to encouraging time out of bed and in a chair for cardiovascular benefit and even short walks in some cases.

Hospital Chaplain

The hospital chaplain is available to provide pastoral care to the critical-care patient, the patient's family members, and staff who may need spiritual support, especially when a patient dies. Chaplains also sometimes get involved in crisis intervention and work closely with social workers to help patients and families cope with the stresses of the ICU environment.

ASKED AND ANSWERED: According to a 2007 survey of fourteen Ontario Hospitals, severely ill women were about one-third less likely to receive treatment in an ICU than were men with comparable conditions. The study, published in the *Canadian Medical Association Journal* concludes that gender bias may be one of the factors responsible for the disparity.

Asking Staff, Informing Family

When your loved one is hovering between life and death in an ICU, or between life and disability, there is no such thing as a wrong or stupid question. Cut yourself some slack—you may be stressed and unable to understand or retain unfamiliar information. Ask anyone on the team about anything you want to know, even down to details that may seem trivial. Ask for an explanation if a response baffles you. Otherwise, team members will assume you have understood. Not sure of what questions to ask? Consult the Questions for ICU Staff quick-reference sheet nearby and at the back of the book. And if you're afraid you won't remember the answers, write them down.

Don't be shy about asking questions on a daily basis. Your loved one's condition can change overnight, and daily discussions with ICU team members allow for updates. If a serious change or event occurs, you may need to speak with the doctor more frequently. The nurses attending your loved one can help keep you updated about the events of the day and can also help clarify information. If multiple doctors are involved, having one of them to speak to the family every day can create a clear channel of communication. Be sure to hold your position as family spokesperson. One doctor representing the ICU side talking with one person representing the family side will help prevent mixed messages. If a difficult decision has to be made or if you're getting unclear information, ask the nurse or the social worker to help convene a family meeting with the doctor. Use the Agenda for a Family Meeting/Conference quick-reference sheet if there's a care issue that you and your family need to discuss with the staff. Call a meeting for all involved, and use the sheet to guide you in the meeting; it's available here in the chapter and with the other tear-out sheets at the back of the book.

If your loved one is not doing well, some members of the immediate family may be tempted to press the clinical team to take aggressive measures. Remember that doctors are not required to offer therapies that they believe won't be medically effective or that they believe won't increase the patient's chances of survival. You may be told that your loved one is not a candidate for certain interventions. If you and your family

Questions for ICU Staff
(Make as many photocopies as you need.)

For the Nurses

Who are the doctors caring for my loved one?

Which doctor is in charge?

Is an intensivist involved in the care of my loved one?

Is there anything in the treatments planned for today that may be painful or uncomfortable?

If so, have medications been ordered to prevent the pain or discomfort?

If you're not in the room, how do I call for help?

How quickly should I expect someone to respond to the call?

How does my loved one go to the bathroom?

Can you explain to me what the doctor said?

Will you explain what all the tubes and equipment are and what they do?

What can I do to help?

What can I do to help my family and myself?

Should I bring anything from home?

Who can visit and when?

If I'm not in the hospital and something happens, how will you get in touch with me?

What happens if something urgent happens and I'm not available?

For the Doctors

What's wrong with my loved one?

Can it be cured?

How will this condition affect my loved one's quality of life?

What's the overall treatment plan?

When do you usually see a response to the treatment or therapy?

What changes will you be watching for as a response to the treatment or therapy?

What are the risks of the therapy and/or medications?

Is my loved one in any pain?

What's being done to ease my loved one's pain and fear?

How is nutrition provided?

Is my loved one receiving the medications to be taken at home?

Notes

disagree with that decision, you can appeal to the hospital ethics committee—the nurse or social worker could tell you how.

Not just immediate family but relatives and friends will be anxious to hear how your loved one is doing. They will want to know what's wrong, how the patient is responding, and what they can do to help. You might be comforted by their concerns, but you might also feel overwhelmed by them—especially in the early days of the crisis. Consider delegating someone in the family to help you field inquiries temporarily, and make sure that person understands what's going on before he or she starts offering explanations to others. You don't want distorted communication, nor do you need free advice from well-intentioned people who don't know what they're talking about. But if friends and relatives can help with needs at home, let them. They will feel better if they can actually do something—both you and the person helping out will benefit.

Some relatives, friends, and colleagues may call the hospital directly to find out how a patient is doing if they don't want to intrude on the family's anxiety. The answers they hear may seem abrupt and even rude. That's because most North American hospitals have now adopted guidelines suggested in 2003 by the American Hospital Association (AHA): standardized one-word descriptions of a patient's condition. The original goal was to help hospitals respond to aggressive media inquiries about patients who were celebrities or public figures. But many hospitals now offer the option to any patient (or substitute decision-maker) so that all general inquiries can receive the same response without violating privacy rules.

The one-word reports are not medical terms. In fact, they are more art than science. They are based on a doctor's best judgment of a patient's condition. Although it is acceptable to use the word *stable* to describe vital signs (blood pressure, pulse, temperature, and respiration), the AHA discourages hospitals from using the word by itself to describe a patient's condition, although it is okay to use it in combination with other words—as in "fair but stable." As one hospital spokesperson put it, "A person can be dead and therefore be stable." The recom-

Agenda for a Family Meeting/Conference
(Make as many photocopies as you need.)

Name of Patient:

Unit and Room Number:

Date and Time of Meeting:

Place of Meeting:

Purpose
    Patient Progress Report:

    Complaint or Conflict (specify):

    Discharge Planning:

    Other (specify):

Family Members Present:

Staff Members Present:

Outcome/Result
    Action Proposed:

    Required Follow-up:

Notes:

mended one-word descriptions are listed here, along with AHA-suggested explanations that may not be provided by the hospital:

UNDETERMINED: Patient awaiting doctor and/or assessment.

GOOD: Vital signs are stable and within normal limits. Patient is conscious and comfortable. Indicators are excellent.

FAIR: Vital signs are stable and within normal limits. Patient is conscious, but may be uncomfortable. Indicators are favorable.

SERIOUS: Vital signs may be unstable and not within normal limits. Patient is acutely ill. Indicators are questionable.

CRITICAL: Vital signs are unstable and not within normal limits. Patient may be unconscious. Indicators are unfavorable.

Not all hospitals follow the AHA recommendations, and some prefer to use their own explanatory language in answering inquiries. For instance, George Washington University Hospital in Washington, DC, defines *critical* as "uncertain prognosis, vital signs are unstable or abnormal, there are major complications, and death may be imminent." Many hospitals add the term "treated and released" to describe patients who received treatment but were not admitted to the hospital. Some hospitals will release news of a death if the family gives permission.

Self-Care in Intensive Care

To be strong for your loved one in the ICU, you have to take care of yourself. That may sound like a platitude, but it's true.

In the early hours or even days of the crisis, you won't want to leave your loved one's side. You will feel worried and helpless and tired, but you'll want to be there all the time in case something, anything, happens. You might fear you could be taking a break at home only to receive a phone call telling you your loved one has died. The impulse to stay and never leave is a natural one. Just be aware that most ICUs will try to discourage you from staying too long, even though ICU visiting schedules are often very relaxed. But some ICUs are starting to offer cots so that a close family member can sleep in the patient's room or cubicle through the deepest parts of a crisis. Many modern ICUs even offer adjacent sleeping facilities for families, with showers, phones, and basic cooking facilities.

Believe that you are as important to the healing process as the doctors and nurses, the medications and treatments. You may have been part of the patient's life for a long time before this crisis. You will be at the hospital whatever happens because you want to be.

Doctors and nurses are finally beginning to acknowledge the strong influence a caring family can have on the healing process. They are learning more and more about the tangible benefits of family involvement in the delivery of patient care; the more enlightened ones will see you as an ally. But they will also worry about you and about the cost to your own health as you cope with a critically ill loved one. And if you're honest, you will probably admit that you're running on adrenalin most of the time.

What is their advice, if you want to remain a useful partner in your loved one's care?

Get proper food and sleep. Both will enhance your ability to listen and absorb the significant clinical information you will be given. Stress is corrosive and can lead to illness. ICU nurses can all tell stories about spouses bedded down in different parts of the same hospital, one being treated in the ICU and the other being treated for exhaustion. Know when to stay and when to go home.

Get up from your loved one's bedside and walk around whenever possible. You've probably known since you were a child that exercise is very important to maintaining emotional health, and the hospital may have some pleasant and distracting outdoor walkways. Find a newspaper and take it with you to the hospital coffee shop or cafeteria—or browse the gift shop. Do you think you're abandoning your loved one? Remember that even experienced ICU doctors and nurses have to take frequent breaks to escape the constant noise and lights and stress.

Try to remain positive. ICU setbacks are fairly common, and they don't necessarily indicate that the patient is in trouble. Remember that recovery from illness never tracks a straight line up. As with life itself, there are peaks and valleys.

Don't feel that you have to be available every minute. A trained medical team is caring for your loved one, and if they know how to find you, they will—fast. Meanwhile, know that your loved one is being closely monitored from the nursing station, even if a nurse isn't next to the bed every single minute.

Book a day off for yourself. Most veteran ICU nurses have uncanny assessment skills, acquired after years of watching for the tiny changes that can signal a shift for the better or the worse in a patient's condition. Pick the most senior nurse you can find who is familiar with your loved one's status, suggest that you might stay away the next day, and ask if that's a good idea. You're not looking for permission—you're consulting an expert. Chances are, you will get a straight answer. Chances are, you can enjoy the respite from a grinding wait. Treat it as your own much-needed recovery time. News is only a phone call away.

6
Recovery (I)
The Ward, the Care Team, and the Plan

Many health-care providers have come to describe the process of recovery as a journey, perhaps to help ease the turmoil, shock, and helplessness generated by injury or illness. The word *journey* seems to suggest hope, purpose, empowerment, and even adventure. It can be an antidote to pessimism and despair.

You may find the metaphor useful to remember on those days when your loved one's journey to recovery feels like a forced and unsettling bus ride, with bounces over potholes, stalls in traffic, and swerves into unexpected detours. There will be stops, too: frequent pauses to admit all kinds of strangers to the bus, who pay close but brief attention to your loved one before hopping off at the next stop, only to be replaced by other strangers who pay close but brief attention to your loved one before hopping off, only to be replaced by other strangers, and then by others, on and on.

In truth, very few patients follow a straight line to recovery, and the major gains are often made in the first few days in the hospital.

At least initially, you and your loved one will probably go to your local community hospital, which is typically defined within the health-care system as an "acute care" hospital. In other words, it was designed to deal with severe illnesses and injuries that can normally be treated over the short term. However, it will also deal with cases that might eventually require specialized or long-term care in another facility.

Milder cases will be treated, too. Patients will not automatically be turned away because their medical needs are not considered serious enough. The "acute care" designation simply describes the ability of the hospital to meet a very wide range of medical challenges. Most people used to call a hospital offering this level of care a general hospital. That was back in the days before hospitals had to work hard to forge close ties to local communities whose goodwill and financial support they now count on.

ASKED AND ANSWERED: There are approximately 7,500 hospitals in the United States and 800 in Canada. The consistent trend in both countries is toward fewer, larger hosptials. The amalgamations are touted as more economically efficient.

According to the American Hospital Association, the average length of stay in a American community hospital was 5.6 days in 2006. Stays have been shortening steadily since 1981, when the average was 7.6 days. An average is fine to know, but it won't tell you exactly how long your loved one will be hospitalized. There are too many variations between individual patients—even those with the same diagnosed condition—for the length of stay to be guaranteed. Recall the "mileage may vary" caution issued by carmakers with gas-economy claims.

The hospital will want to free up your loved one's bed as soon as possible (without being outright reckless) both because someone else will probably be waiting for it and because accountants are knocking on the door. Shorter hospital stays are the result of significant medical advances—hospitals can now cure many conditions more quickly than used to be possible—and also the result of constant pressure to cut climbing health-care costs by reducing length of stays while avoiding any risk of harm to patients. But in 2000 researchers at the University of Michigan studied the accounting records of more than twelve thousand patients and concluded that shorter hospital stays result in minimal savings. In fact, the first few days consume the most resources, and the final day consumes only 3.4 percent of the total cost of the patient's care.

Not only are recovering patients being released from the hospital sooner than they used to be, but all kinds of treatments that once required hospitalization are now becoming widely accepted on an outpatient basis. Day surgeries are popular with both hospitals and the public because they involve only a few hours in a clinic. The trend is being hailed as win-win: patients are being treated faster and going home faster (where they will presumably be happier), and a stressed health-care system is saving money. What could be better?

Watch and Learn

The crowd-pleasing speed and efficiency comes at a cost. The accelerated discharge of patients from the hospital imposes a burden on the very people who are usually kept out of the clinical loop while their loved one is in the hospital. These relatives and friends aren't taught the basics of patient care, but they are expected to pick up the slack after the patient leaves the hospital. That's why one of your tasks as a caregiver at your loved one's side in the hospital is to watch and learn.

Start by paying close attention while your loved one is being "settled in." Settling in is the formal ritual that follows a patient's admission to a ward in the hospital where the sick and the injured are tended until they are judged well enough to go home. Patients may be admitted to the ward after an emergency illness or injury, or they may be transferred there from an ICU or a post-operation recovery room. Transfers are often based on bed availability. They normally happen quickly and without notice, prompted by another patient's need to be in the ICU or recovery room. They are also prompted by a patient's condition, if it is considered stable enough for the patient to be moved to a ward and a bed is now available there.

SMART MOVES: **Settling In**

- Plan to be present for your loved one's transfer to a hospital ward. Be aware that your loved one may become confused or disoriented by the shift from an environment with close nursing care to one where she or he may share a nurse with as many as twelve other patients. There will be a period of adjustment.
- Make sure any personal belongings (glasses, hairbrush, toothbrush, etc.) travel with your loved one to the ward.
- Offer to help move your loved one from the gurney to the bed in the ward and introduce yourself to the nurses helping out.
- Spend some time helping your loved one get comfortable with the new surroundings. Even the bed itself may be different from the specialized-care variations used in the ICU or the post-operation recovery room.
- Notice how the nurses move the patient, adjust the bed, and generally attend to the patient. You may eventually be doing the same things yourself.

Location, Location, Location

Not just your loved one but you yourself will need time to adjust to the hospital ward. If your loved one has been moved from a unit where he or she was alone in the room, you may be blinking your eyes and looking around at as many as three other patients in a shared room—and with only curtains to separate the beds. There goes personal privacy.

Once settled in, your loved one may be ready for a short nap. This could be your opportunity to withdraw for a few minutes and take a quick tour of the ward and your routes beyond it.

As you stroll the hallway, you may pass as many as thirty rooms housing patients with a variety of conditions. Depending on the hospital, the rooms may be classed as standard (four patients per room), semiprivate (two patients per room), or private (one patient per room). Patients or their families are encouraged to request any type of accommodation they want before admission, but most public or private insurers will cover only the costs of a standard room unless there are valid clinical grounds for isolation or privacy. Semiprivate and private rooms are assigned at the discretion of the hospital anyway, and the supply is usually limited. Even if you're prepared to pay extra for a private room, one may not be available.

Locate the nursing station. It's the nerve center of the ward. During business hours a clerk is usually on duty to answer questions and offer assistance with everything from organizing an extra-cost phone or television for a patient's room to helping to locate the doctor responsible for a patient's care. Patients' medical charts are stored at the nursing station, and nurses gather there to make chart entries, trade care notes on patients, organize medications and dressings, and discuss patient assignments.

Locate yourself. This may sound odd, but you could get lost easily, despite excellent signage and even clever color-coded directional lines painted on floors or walls. Most hospitals of any age started with one building and added more over succeeding decades. Some hospitals look like a jumble of blocks bolted together by catwalks, and the blocks don't seem to have any architectural relationship with one another. Worse, hospital expansion is often ongoing, so detours are common. You may wish for a GPS to find your loved one—but all you really need to know are the wing, the floor number, and the room number. Ask the nursing station clerk if a hospital map is available. If not, go exploring and rack up a series of personal mental markers that can serve as your own version of dropping bread crumbs behind you in the woods.

If you want a record of where you are, as well as other numbers and names, fill out the Handy Hospital Information quick-reference sheet at the back of the book, tear it out, and carry it with you. That way, if you get lost, you will at least be able to ask for directions back. (You can also find the information form nearby in this chapter.)

Locate the family lounge. It can be a separate room or an alcove, typically furnished with comfortable chairs and perhaps a vending machine or two, as well as a television set—one that seems to be on twenty-four hours a day. A visit to a nearby family lounge can give you a quick break from the bedside, and the lounge can also serve as an informal gathering place for conversations with family and friends.

Handy Hospital Information
(Make as many photocopies as you need.)

Name and Address of Hospital:

Key Hospital Phone Numbers:

  Patient:

  General Inquiries:

  Patient Inquiries:

  Patient Relations:

  Billing/Accounts Inquiries:

  Executive Offices:

Patient's Location (wing, floor, room number):

Name of Attending Physician:

  Pager Number:

Name of Charge Nurse:

  Nursing Station Direct Line:

Notes

Locate the elevator bank that serves the ward. You will want to know how to find your loved one's room efficiently after arriving—and how to leave when you're ready to go home at night.

Check out hospital resources that can help you take an occasional break without straying too far from your loved one's bedside. Most lobbies have turned into mini-malls that include a coffee shop or two, a convenience store with a magazine rack, a drugstore, a gift shop, and one or two public seating areas. If you're hungry, the self-serve hospital cafeteria is a good bet for simple meals. Since it is also used by hospital staff, you may find yourself sharing a table with a top surgeon or a hospital executive, not to mention other patients' families. Let someone at the nursing station know where you are and roughly how long you will be away so you can be found in a hurry if needed. Make a list of nearby getaway possibilities and other hospital resources on the Caregiver Resources at the Hospital quick-reference sheet at the back of the book and carry it with you (the sheet is also printed nearby).

The Recovery-Ward Care Team

Now that you've figured out exactly where you are, you can begin to get a sense of the people responsible for your loved one's care. The membership of recovery-ward care teams varies from hospital to hospital, but a typical one could include the following professionals.

Attending Doctor

An attending doctor (often called the staff doctor) leads the team and has been assigned overall responsibility for your loved one's care in the hospital. Along with residents (see below), the attending doctor examines your loved one, monitors daily progress, plans overall care, and oversees treatment. The attending doctor also maintains close contact with your family doctor. If so-called hospital privileges have been granted to your family doctor, he or she will be welcome to drop in and see how your loved one is doing.

Caregiver Resources at the Hospital
(Make as many photocopies as you need.)

"I need a short break."
Location of Nearest Visitors' Lounge:

Couch or Cot Available?

TV or Music Available?

Internet Connectivity Available?

Location of Nearest Book/Magazine Shop:

Location of Nearest Coffee Shop:

Location of Hospital Cafeteria: Hours Open:

Location of Shower Facilities:

Location of Hospital Chapel:

Location of Nearby Places to Stroll (landscaped hospital grounds, parks, shops):

"I need help resolving some questions and concerns."
Location of Patient Relations Office:

Name of Person in Charge:

Name of Social Worker:

Phone and Pager Numbers:

Name of Chaplain:

   Phone and Pager Numbers:

"Family are arriving, and we need a private place to talk."
Location of Nearest Family Room or Lounge:

Date and Time of Reservation:

Name and Title of Person Available to Answer Family's Questions:

   Phone and Pager Numbers:

Location of Nearby Hotel/Motel Accommodations:

Hospitalist

Some hospitals are now employing hospitalists, a new kind of doctor who provides care to patients all the way from admission right through to discharge. They are a boon to patients who don't have a family doctor. But those who do will not normally see their family doctor until after they leave the hospital. Hospitalists are completely in charge of their patients from admission forward, and only courtesy compels them to update the family doctor. Unlike many other doctors in the hospital, they don't maintain offices off-site. Unlike family doctors, they work regular hours and are seldom on call. Hospitalists undergo additional training in case management, and many of them are specialists in internal medicine, with supplementary roles in staff education.

ASKED AND ANSWERED: The word *hospitalist* did not exist before 1996. Currently, only about 40 percent of U.S. hospitals have hospitalists.

Consultants

Consultants are doctors with acknowledged expertise in particular areas. The attending doctor or hospitalist may call them in to assist with diagnosis and treatment of a particular clinical condition by asking for a "consult"—shorthand for a consultation. Among the consultants who can be summoned to the patient's bedside are those with the following specialties. The name of the particular kind of specialist is in parentheses.

> *Allergy and Immunology (allergist-immunologist)*—Diagnosis and treatment of problems involving the immune system, including allergic reactions to foods, drugs, chemicals, insect stings, and pollens. Allergic conditions include hay fever, asthma, hives, dermatitis, eczema, and acquired immune deficiency diseases.

Anesthesia (anesthetist or anesthesiologist)—The administering of drugs called anesthetics for relief of pain during surgery. The anesthetist may use a local or a regional anesthetic, including a spinal or an epidural anesthetic, which dulls sensation in a part of the body, or a general anesthetic, which renders a patient unconscious.

Cardiology (cardiologist)—Diagnosis and treatment of diseases of the heart and blood vessels, such as heart attacks and life-threatening abnormal heartbeats. Diagnostic procedures include interpretation of electrocardiograms and echocardiograms and supervision of and interpretation of stress tests and cardiac catheterization. The cardiologist evaluates the need for cardiac surgery.

Dermatology (dermatologist)—Diagnosis and treatment of benign and malignant disorders of the skin, mouth, external genitalia, hair, and nails. Skin cancers, melanomas, moles, and other tumors of the skin, as well as contact dermatitis and other manifestations of systemic infectious diseases, are treated. The specialty also includes management of cosmetic disorders of the skin, such as hair loss and scars. Treatment methods include medications that are externally applied, injected, or taken orally; selected X-ray and ultraviolet-light therapy; and surgery.

Endocrinology (endocrinologist)—Evaluation and treatment of disorders of the internal glands, such as the thyroid and adrenal glands; also of disorders such as diabetes, metabolic and nutritional disorders, pituitary diseases, and menstrual and sexual problems. A subspecialty of internal medicine.

Gastroenterology (gastroenterologist)—Management and treatment of disorders associated with the digestive organs, including the stomach, bowel, liver, and gallbladder. Abdominal pain, ulcers, diarrhea, rectal bleeding, cancer, and jaundice are also treated. Lighted scopes (endoscopes) are used to see internal organs for diagnostic and therapeutic procedures. When abdominal operations are indicated, a gastroenterologist will consult with a surgeon. A subspecialty of internal medicine.

Geriatric Medicine, Gerontology (gerontologist)—The prevention, diagnosis, and treatment of diseases and disorders of the elderly, including comprehensive care management of patients with multiple disabilities, such as dementia, diabetes, cerebrovascular and cardiovascular conditions, osteoporosis, and arthritis.

Hospital Medicine (hospitalist)—A new branch of medicine organized around a site of care (the hospital), rather than an organ or a disease. Unlike other specialists, hospitalists will often see patients in the emergency department and stay with them all the way to recovery, providing an important continuum of care. Depending on the hospital, the specialty may also include teaching and research. A majority of hospitalists are trained in internal medicine.

Hematology (hematologist)—Diagnosis and treatment of hematologic (blood) malignancies, including Hodgkin's disease, non-Hodgkin's lymphomas, myeloproliferative disorders, myelodysplastic syndromes, and leukemias. Also, diagnosis and treatment of nonmalignant hematologic disorders, including anemia, thalassemias, clotting disorders, sickle cell disease, and hemophilia.

Infectious Disease (internist)—Diagnosis and treatment of infectious diseases of all types, including treatment of patients with HIV infection and AIDS. Diagnosis and management of unusual infections and unexplained fevers. A subspecialty of internal medicine.

Internal Medicine (internist)—Diagnosis and comprehensive care management of internal illnesses and problems, as well as management of preventive health care and wellness. Also, management of heart disease, diabetes, and lung and digestive diseases. Also, travel medicine, including consultation and vaccinations. There are many subspecialties within internal medicine.

Nephrology (nephrologist)—Diagnosis and treatment of disorders of the kidney and related body fluid and chemical imbalances. A nephrologist is responsible for administering dialysis when the kidneys do not function and for providing advice to surgeons about kidney transplants. A subspecialty of internal medicine.

Neurology (neurologist)—Diagnosis and treatment of disorders of the peripheral and central nervous systems, including their supporting structures and blood vessels. Strokes, epilepsy, multiple sclerosis, and spinal cord disorders are typical problems that are treated and diagnosed.

Obstetrics and Gynecology (obstetrician-gynecologist, or ob-gyn, pronounced "o-b-g-y-n")—Specialty in the female reproductive system and/or the fetus and the newborn. Obstetrics involves care of women during pregnancy, delivery of babies, and follow-up treatment. Gynecology is the diagnosis and treatment of disorders of the female reproductive organs and the reproductive process, including infertility, infections of the genital tract, cancer of the genital organs, and complications of pregnancy. Pelvic surgeries, including hysterectomies, are performed.

Oncology (oncologist)—Diagnosis and treatment of tumors, including lung, breast, colon, rectum, anus, small bowel, liver, biliary system, pancreas, stomach, esophagus, kidney, bladder, prostate, testes, uterus, ovary, cervix, skin, and head and neck cancers.

Ophthalmology (ophthalmologist)—Diagnosis and treatment of disorders of the eye, including glaucoma. Also, vision care, including comprehensive eye examinations and prescriptions for eyeglasses and contact lenses. Ophthalmologists perform surgery to repair such ailments as cataracts and retinal detachments; also nearsightedness and astigmatism. They may also detect disease in other parts of the body through eye examination—for example, diabetes, thyroid disease, brain tumors, and hypertension (high blood pressure).

Orthopedic Surgery (orthopedic surgeon)—Diagnosis and treatment of bones, joints, and muscles. Treatment of injuries, disorders, and diseases related to the function of the extremities, the spine, and associated structures by surgical and physical procedures. Diagnosis and treatment of congenital deformities, trauma, infections, tumors, and metabolic disturbances of the muscular and skeletal systems. Treatment may involve arthroscopic examinations (of joints using a surgically inserted fiber-optic instrument) and surgery of the joints.

Otolaryngology; Ear, Nose, and Throat, or ENT (otolaryngologist; ear, nose, and throat doctor)—Diagnosis and medical and surgical treatment of diseases and disorders of the ear, nose, and throat, respiratory and upper alimentary systems, and related structures. Also, evaluation and treatment of hearing. Head and neck oncology sometimes is involved, as is plastic and reconstructive surgery of the face. The specialty includes knowledge of audiology and speech-language pathology.

Pathology (pathologist)—The diagnosis of disease through the study of body tissues, secretions. and fluids. Includes use of scientific instruments and analytical measurements and procedures. A pathologist examines tissues and blood chemically and microscopically to arrive at a diagnosis.

Physical Medicine and Rehabilitation (physiatrist)—Evaluation and supervised treatment of impairments caused by stroke, arthritis, head injury, spinal cord injury, multiple sclerosis, Parkinson's disease, and cerebral palsy. Includes pain management, disability evaluations, and adjunctive treatment following orthopedic procedures or surgery. Treatment may involve use of therapeutic heat, cold, massage, ultrasound, electrical stimulation, exercise, and mechanical devices and prosthetics. A physiatrist often approves a rehabilitation program and directs the work of physical therapists (in Canada: physiotherapists).

Plastic Surgery (plastic surgeon)—Surgery to correct functional and cosmetic deformities of the face, head, body, and extremities. A plastic surgeon repairs scarred or burned skin, reconstructs structures destroyed by cancer or accidents, and performs surgery to correct congenital abnormalities or to improve the appearance of a part of the body. The specialty includes cosmetic surgery and surgery related to reconstruction; breast reduction and breast lift; head and neck cancer; skin cancer, including melanomas; hand surgery; cleft lip and palate surgery; eyelid ptosis surgery; maxillo-facial surgery; reconstructive nasal surgery; body contouring (lipo-suction, tummy tucks, etc.); and management of open or chronic wounds, including pressure sores and leg ulcers.

Podiatry (podiatrist)—Diagnosis and treatment of diseases and disorders of the foot, including soft tissue disorders such as corns, bunions, and ingrown toenails. Podiatrists may specialize in podi-atric surgery.

Psychiatry (psychiatrist)—Prevention, diagnosis, and treatment of mental and emotional disorders, including depression, anxiety dis-orders, substance abuse, developmental disabilities, and sexual dysfunctions. Treatment includes psychotherapy, psychoanalysis, laboratory diagnostic tests, medications, and intervention with in-dividuals and families who are coping with stress, crisis, and other emotional problems. Subspecializations exist in child, adolescent, and geriatric psychiatry.

Psychology (psychologist)—Evaluation, diagnosis, and treatment of mental, emotional, and behavioral disorders and discomforts. Treatment typically involves counseling and psychotherapy. Un-like a psychiatrist, a psychologist is not authorized to admit a pa-tient to the hospital.

Pulmonary Medicine (pulmonist); in Canada: Respirology (respir-ologist)—Diagnosis and treatment of diseases and disorders of the lungs and airways. Includes such conditions as pneumonia, cancer, pleurisy, asthma, bronchitis, and emphysema. Tests may include measurement of breathing volume, bronchoscopy, and X-rays. Treatment involves administering drugs, mechanical assistance in breathing, and consultation with surgeons. A subspecialty of inter-nal medicine.

Radiology (radiologist)—The use of various methods, such as X-rays, mammography, ultrasound, magnetic resonance imaging (MRI), CT (CAT) scans, and nuclear medicine, to diagnose and treat disease. Specialties include radiation oncology, diagnostic ra-diology, and nuclear medicine.

Respirology (respirologist)—*See* Pulmonary Medicine

Rheumatology (rheumatologist)—Diagnosis and nonsurgical treatment of diseases of the joints, muscle, bones, and tendons, including such conditions as arthritis, back pains, muscle strains, and collagen diseases. A subspecialty of internal medicine.

Surgery (surgeon)—The preoperative, operative, and postoperative care of patients treated for a broad span of surgical conditions affecting most areas of the body. Can involve comprehensive management of a trauma victim or the critically ill. There are many subspecialties of surgery.

Urology (urologist)—Treatment of diseases of the urinary tract of both males and females and of the reproductive system of the male. The organs treated include the kidneys, bladder, prostate gland, adrenal gland, penis, and testes. Diagnostic procedures include examination of urine samples, X-rays, ultrasound, and use of the cystoscope. The conditions treated through medication, surgery, and/or minimally invasive surgical techniques include bladder infections, incontinence, impotency, male infertility, kidney infections, kidney stones, prostate enlargements, and benign and malignant tumors of the urinary tract and prostate gland.

Residents

Residents are licensed doctors receiving additional specialty training at the hospital. During their residency program, they provide care under the supervision of an attending doctor.

Fellows

Fellows are licensed doctors who have completed a residency program and are now receiving advanced training in a specialty.

Physician Assistants

Physician assistants are health professionals licensed to practice medicine under the supervision of a doctor. They make medical decisions and provide a broad range of diagnostic and therapeutic services.

Nurses

Several types of nurse may be involved in your loved one's care.

Charge nurses (also called nurse managers; formerly called head nurses)—Charge nurses are responsible for the overall leadership of the ward. They are a valuable resource for patients and families who need help resolving problems or addressing concerns.

Registered nurses (RNs)—Registered nurses provide direct care to patients and observe, assess, and record symptoms, reactions, and progress. They also assist doctors during treatments and examinations, administer medications, and assist in convalescence and rehabilitation, as well as educate patients and their families.

Licensed practical nurses (LPNs); in Canada: registered practical nurses (RPNs)—These nurses are assigned to particular patients each shift and assist the registered nurses in performing clinical tasks.

Advanced registered nurse practitioners; in Canada: advanced practice nurses—These are registered nurses with additional education and clinical training in a specific area of health care. There are several kinds of advanced registered nurse practitioners, including clinical nurse specialists (who specialize in one area of nursing) and nurse practitioners (who perform physical examinations, diagnose patient problems, treat illness, educate patients and families, and participate in research programs).

Respiratory Therapists

Respiratory therapists evaluate and treat patients with breathing problems. They provide oxygen and other therapies, monitor ventilators (respirators), and offer education and equipment to patients who need ongoing respiratory care beyond the hospital stay.

Pharmacists

Acting on clinical orders, pharmacists prepare and dispense medications. They work closely with doctors and nurses to monitor drug therapies and to prevent or correct drug interactions. They will answer questions that you may have about your loved one's prescribed medications and discuss potential side effects.

Dietitians

Dietitians are nutrition experts who evaluate and modify a patient's eating patterns. They work with family and medical staff to recommend dietary changes that will promote recovery and prevent complications.

Physical Therapists (in Canada: Physiotherapists)

Physical therapists evaluate the patient's developmental and functional skills. They treat physical, developmental, and neurological problems and help patients achieve mobility through customized rehabilitation programs.

Occupational Therapists

Occupational therapists assess motor, sensory, cognitive, perceptual, and psychosocial development. Based on assessments, they help patients gain maximum independence through routine activities like dressing, bathing, and eating that help define a person's normal day.

Social Workers

Social workers assist families with emotional, physical, and financial concerns related to the patient's illness. They're on standby to help during hospitalization and discharge. Social workers refer families to financial and social service resources and coordinate with community and educational agencies near the patient's home.

Medical Students

If the hospital is a teaching facility, medical students might be present from time to time to observe and learn. They often participate in care while holding to the same standards of patient confidentiality and practice as staff do.

Key Members of the Team You Should Get to Know

Know the Attending Doctor or Hospitalist

Most hospital doctors are terrible communicators. They may have taken a quick course on talking to patients and families in medical school, but they are scientists at core, and their primary interest is usually clinical. The patient's relatives will be treated with respect but will also be considered peripheral at this stage in the treatment and recovery process. What's more, in the hospital setting your loved one may be only one of dozens of patients they are responsible for; they usually spend their days racing from one room to the next. That said, you can possibly strike up a relationship that establishes your willingness to assist in care. You can at least make sure you're in their field of vision—and that you get the essential clinical information you need to be useful at your loved one's bedside. If you have questions for the doctor, write them down—and then write down the answers. Be confident enough to ask for elaboration on any points you didn't understand.

Know the Charge Nurse

The charge nurse has a wide array of management duties, which range from assigning and scheduling nurses to overseeing the complete care of every patient on the ward. He or she will be the go-to person if you have any questions or concerns about your loved one's care that cannot be resolved by the nurse looking after your loved one. Most charge nurses make a habit of visiting every patient every day and receive regular briefings on patient status from the nursing staff; some of them even pitch in to help with direct patient care when needed. They may be authorized to call for consultations without permission from the attending doctor. They will also order special beds or supplies, assist with discharge planning, share test results with you, deal with any conflicts you may have with staff, and support your efforts to help by offering suggestions and comments.

Know the Other Nurses

The nurses providing direct care to your loved one all once wanted to be Florence Nightingale. They wanted to be as tough and compassionate and idealistic. They were as driven to make a real difference as their legendary predecessor. But the hectic world of twenty-first-century nursing seldom gives them a chance to fulfill their earliest hopes. Twelve-hour shifts and high patient ratios have become the norm, and nurses in modern hospitals often spend their days in a grinding routine of complex tasks that make them slaves to the clock. Along the way, they endure abusive patients unconsciously seeking an outlet for their own frustration, families who expect them to come running when the call bell sounds, and doctors who behave like high-handed aristocrats dealing with a lower class.

ASKED AND ANSWERED: There are about 2,400,000 registered nurses in the United States (U.S. Census Bureau; 2005) and about 252,000 in Canada (Canadian Institute for Health Information; 2006), with an average age of forty-five in both countries. The totals are shrinking annually as nurses continue to quit the profession or retire. Even with evidence of increased enrollment in nursing schools, it's expected that demand will exceed supply by 2020.

Surprisingly, very few veteran nurses are hardened and cynical. Most remain empathetic and deeply committed. Note their names and remember them. Be ready to share some personal details of your family—some of the life you and your loved one enjoy outside the hospital—and to listen to them talk about theirs. Conversations like that can help turn your relationship with them from merely cordial to therapeutic for everyone and cement a beneficial partnership. Nurses can become your closest allies in your loved one's care and sometimes respond with touching gratitude to a late-afternoon cup of coffee or snack that you've brought from the hospital coffee shop. Once they are comfortable with you, most will gladly accept offers of help at the bedside.

Generally, doctors bring their minds to their care challenges, but nurses also bring their hearts. That can often make the difference between basic recovery and whole-person healing.

Know the Dietitians

Your loved one may be a finicky eater at the best of times, and a hospital stay isn't the best time. He or she may not have much interest in eating at first, and although hospital food is a common target of unfair criticism, most hospital dietitians are happy to work with families toward providing food that's both nutritious and enjoyable. They will also need to be aware of any food allergies your loved one may have, as well as any dietary restrictions because of religious or other beliefs—they will need to know, for example, if your loved one is a vegetarian. Identifying the right food may be a trial-and-error challenge that will take time and patience. You can always ask the dietitian if a favorite choice from home might help kick-start your loved one's appetite.

Know the Physical Therapists (Physiotherapists) and Occupational Therapists

Muscles weaken after surgery or the onset of a serious illness amazingly quickly, even in people who pumped iron or ran marathons before the crisis. At some point, when your loved one needs to start moving again, she or he will undergo assessment by physical therapists and occupational therapists, who will design programs with restored mobility as the goal. Because you know your loved one, you can be useful in a variety of ways—from sharing some of your loved one's interests with therapists to cheering your loved one through what will undoubtedly be a tedious series of repetitive moves. Many hospitals discourage family members from being present for physical therapy sessions, but exceptions are made, and if you've demonstrated your willingness to help, there's a good chance you will be welcome.

The Care Plan

Care planning is an essential part of health care, although it is often misunderstood or even dismissed in some places as a waste of time. Clinical experts argue, however, that without a specific document outlining the plan of care, important issues can be neglected.

A care plan is essentially a road map for the journey of recovery. It guides everyone involved in the patient's care. But to assume that nurses have the sole responsibility for implementing it shortchanges the other members of the care team, implicitly assigning them a secondary role. The assumption also overloads the nurses, imposing unfair responsibilities on them. Any effective and comprehensive care plan should bring all the members of the care team on board, not to mention the patient's family.

Care plans are developed in stages. The first step is an accurate and comprehensive patient assessment, which provides a clinical baseline on which to build the plan. The assessment is usually undertaken by nurses working with the attending doctor when your loved one is admitted to the recovery ward, and it includes all the clinical information about your loved one to that point. A good care plan is flexible: it allows for changes. The initial assessment is usually followed by scheduled reassessments during your loved one's hospital stay.

Let's say the diagnosis is severe pneumonia. Even a fairly common condition like that comes with its own set of ancillary problems, which are carefully listed in the initial assessment. The assessment could also include a list of the patient's physical strengths and weaknesses and observed or known information about family or relationship tensions that might affect the patient's well-being. The ideal care plan takes into account all of the variables—physical as well as psychological—that might have an impact on recovery.

In reviewing the list of problems, members of the care team are encouraged to ask a simple question about each one: "Can we make this problem go away?" If the answer is yes, and if appropriate medications and therapies are agreed on, then everyone's aim is to see the problem diminish within a designated period of time—the next day or the next week or the next month. Improvement goals should be specific, measurable, and attainable. For instance, the ideal care plan will not vaguely predict that a bedsore "will be improved by next week." That is not useful. Given the slow and erratic recovery rate of most bedsores, that goal is probably not attainable either. A better goal statement would be explicit, taking into account the precise physical dimensions of the wound and projecting measurable improvement over a reasonable time period.

If a problem isn't likely to diminish or go away, then an effective care plan will address how to keep it from worsening. Diabetes and congestive heart failure are examples—they can't be cured, but they can be managed. The care plan should include specific measures to prevent or minimize complications or deterioration, with measurable goal statements about maintaining blood sugar and blood pressure within specific limits.

Sometimes problems cannot be effectively managed. Deterioration is inevitable for patients with Alzheimer's, for instance, but there is still a need for a care plan. It might include strategies for providing comfort and preserving the patient's dignity, and it might list medications and treatments that will help delay complications and decline. The goal is to provide optimal quality of life within the limits of the disease. For someone with dementia, one written goal statement might be to help the patient maintain the ability to recognize family members and participate in simple yes/no daily decision-making until the next review date.

Care plans vary from hospital to hospital. Some are overseen and directed by doctors, some result from established hospital protocol, and some are just accepted medical practice. Some hospitals may require that medication dosages and times be spelled out in the care plan, while others may endorse a more general approach by simply encouraging clinical staff to comply with formal doctors' orders. Whichever the approach, a care plan is invariably included in the patient's official record, or medical chart—normally called the chart by hospital staff—while your loved one is hospitalized. There's more about the chart and its important role in documenting each patient's care history in the next chapter.

The best care plans are fluid and adaptable. They allow for setbacks as well as improvements in the status of the patient, and they remain active until the patient is discharged. They are reviewed and updated regularly as problems resolve and the patient's condition improves. Ideally, a detailed care plan read by anyone tending your loved one will immediately provide all the information needed for whole-person care to continue.

An example of a care plan notable for its clarity and orderly progression is included here courtesy of the Alberta Bone and Joint Health Institute. It is a care plan for a patient having a total knee replacement, but the basic form could be used for anyone under hospital care.

SMART MOVES: **Working with the Care Plan**

- Ask the attending doctor or charge nurse for the details and goals of your loved one's care plan and transcribe them for yourself.

- Once you've reviewed the plan, identify any elements that you believe might be inappropriate for your loved one (such as dietary recommendations or medications) and immediately voice your concerns to the attending doctor or charge nurse.

- Look for opportunities within the care plan to get actively involved in care, from medical treatments and tests to physical or occupational therapy.

- Immediately report any unusual physical or psychological responses by your loved one. They could reflect a subtle but important negative reaction to drugs or therapies.

- Ask for a care plan review if you have concerns or questions, and ask if goals are being met.

Total Knee Replacement Patient Care Plan

Care	Day of Surgery	Day 1 Post-Op
Nutrition	Intravenous (IV) started for fluids and medications Catheter may be inserted in bladder; urine output monitored for 24 hours	Fluids taken as tolerated Sit up for meals as able IV as needed Catheter removed Start bowel routine Go to bathroom by commode chair/walker with help
Hygiene	Assisted mouth and skin care as needed	Wash at sink or basin
Wound Care	Dressing checked and changed or reinforced as needed	Wound checked daily Dressing removed and wound redressed if draining
Pain Control/ Medication	IV or oral medications for pain control once spinal wears off May have epidural (local anaesthetic)	IV or oral pain medication continued Patient asks for pain medication when needed
Activity/ Rehab	Patient does the following exercises every hour after surgery when awake: • Deep breathing and coughing • Foot and ankle exercises Do not rest knee in bent position on pillow Sit up on side of bed and stand with help Walk if able and as requested by doctor	Deep breathing and coughing Transfer to/from bed and chair with help Sit up in chair for short periods Walk using walker/crutches with help (not exceeding doctor-ordered weight limit on operated leg) Begin daily rehab to increase range of motion and exercises to strengthen operated leg

Total Knee Replacement Patient Care Plan (continued)

Care	Day of Surgery	Day 1 Post-Op
Discharge Planning	Expected length of stay is 3–4 days Planned day of discharge is written on bedside communication board	Patient discusses discharge needs (i.e. equipment, services) with care providers

Care	Day 2 Post-Op	Days 3–4 Post-Op
Nutrition	Diet as tolerated Sit up in chair for all meals Discontinue IV if no nausea and no IV medications needed	Sit up in chair for all meals Enema or suppository given if no bowel movement
Hygiene		Shower if able
Wound Care	Dressing removed and wound redressed if draining	Incision exposed when wound is dry
Pain Control/ Medication	Pain medication taken as needed and coordinated with activity or rehabilitation schedule	Pain control medication taken prior to exercise Patient reviews home instructions for giving self anti-coagulant to help prevent blood clotting
Activity/ Rehab	Deep breathing and coughing Increase frequency of transfers to/from bed and chair, and increase independence of transfers Increase distance and frequency of walks, and progress to crutches as able Continue exercises (with therapist and independently)	Deep breathing and coughing Progress to crutches as appropriate Review procedure for going up and down stairs Review home exercises Continue to increase independent transfers to/from bed and chair and walking to bathroom and in hallway as able

Total Knee Replacement Patient Care Plan (continued)

Care	Day 2 Post-Op	Days 3–4 Post-Op
	Occupational therapy initiated as needed	Attend physiotherapy session Attend occupational therapy session to review tub transfers and dressing if needed
Discharge Planning	Nurse, physio and occupational therapists confirm discharge plan and equipment in place Resources contacted as needed (i.e. sub-acute facility, Home Care, mobile lab)	Out-patient physiotherapy arranged if requested by surgeon (when new knee has less than 70° of flexion and/or thigh muscles significantly weak)

Care	Discharge Goals
Nutrition	Eating and bowel movements returning to normal
Hygiene	Able to manage personal hygiene without help
Wound Care	Surgical wound is clean and dry, or wound care management arranged for home Removal of staples or stitches arranged
Pain Control/ Medication	Pain management discussed with and understood by patient Required prescriptions provided to patient
Activity/ Rehab	Patient is able to: • Achieve minimum 70° flexion in operated leg • Transfer to/from bed and chair and stand independently and safely • Walk 30 metres using walking aid without exceeding doctor-ordered weight limit on operated leg • Go up and down stairs safely • Perform home exercises and daily living activities safely (or has support in place at home for required activities)

Discharge Goals (continued)

	Patient will be transferred to sub-acute facility if more rehab needed
Discharge Planning	Patient is given and understands: • Discharge instructions • Required exercise routine • Follow-up appointment dates

Source: Reproduced by permission from the Alberta Bone and Joint Health Institute, 2008. Graphics are omitted.

7
Recovery (II)
Charts, Meds, Tests, Codes, and
Other Hospital Mysteries

The professionals around you in the hospital are always consulting it and talking about it. Their murmured comments range from enthusiastic to worried, and you overhear two staff members vigorously discussing what various inscriptions mean and how they should be altered or updated. Pages are added. People pause to scribble in it or spend long periods studying it. Depending on the hospital and the severity of your loved one's condition, it may reside on a table close to the bed. You're curious, but you're not allowed to read it.

What is it? A medical chart. Every hospital patient has one. A confidential document, the chart serves as both a medical and a legal record of the patient's clinical care from admission to discharge. By detailing diagnoses, treatments, medications, test results, and other significant information, the hospital staff who make and update the chart entries share with their colleagues everything they know about the patient's ongoing clinical condition. It's an efficient go-to resource for all the people looking after your loved one.

Health-care providers treat each patient's medical chart as a sacred trust, and that's why you aren't permitted access to it without the patient's express permission, no matter how close you and the patient may be. But it's important to understand its central role in care, and it could even be worth replicating in your own way.

The Medical Chart

Although most charts are still loose-leaf binders that can weigh more than a big-city phone book, depending on the patient's length of stay and the complexity of the illness, some hospitals are now using computers for entering information. The advantages are legible, organized documentation, enhanced access, and efficient storage. The major disadvantage is that some of these electronic records are vulnerable to being hacked by any computer-smart fifteen-year-old. But hospitals are very sensitive to the need for confidentiality, and most can outrun cyberspace intruders with anti-hacking software that is continually improved.

Even within the hospital, access to the chart is limited to authorized personnel. Doctors and nurses are the most frequent users. Doctors make regular entries about diagnoses and prognoses as well as treatment recommendations. Nurses record patient responses to treatments and details of day-to-day progress. In many hospitals, doctors and nurses use separate forms or areas of the chart specific to their disciplines.

Other on-staff health-care professionals who have legitimate reasons to make entries in the chart include physician assistants, psychiatrists, social workers, psychologists, dietitians, physical and occupational therapists, respiratory therapists, and consultants. Everyone is encouraged to read everyone else's entries so that each has a complete clinical profile of the patient, making continuity of care possible. In some jurisdictions, quality-assurance and regulatory organizations, legal agencies, and insurance companies may also have access to the chart for specific purposes such as documentation, institutional audits, legal proceedings, or verification of information for care reimbursement. That opens the chart to more eyes, making confidentiality even more important.

While the patient is in the hospital, the chart is often stored in a secure area like the nursing station for easy access by clinicians. It is discussed only in appropriate and private clinical areas—not in the hallway, for instance. Every patient has the right to view and obtain copies of his or her medical record, and special state and provincial statutes cover sensitive information—for example, psychiatric evaluations, confirming tests for communicable diseases, and substance abuse records. Institutional and government policies control what is contained in the chart and how it is documented—and there are rules governing access to the chart that also protect its integrity and confidentiality. When chart contents need to be accessed by people outside the hospital, the patient or the patient's representative is asked for written permission to release records. Patients are also often asked to sign releases when they are transferred out of the hospital so that caregivers in new clinical settings can review their charts.

What's in the Chart?

The process of building the medical chart starts as soon as a patient enters the hospital for care. Hospitals often request permission to obtain copies of previous health records so that they have complete information on the patient from the beginning. Although chart systems might vary from institution to institution, most elements are universal. They are typically organized into sections, including these:

ADMISSION PAPERWORK: Legal paperwork, including a living will or health-care proxy; the patient's demographic profile; and contact information.

HISTORY AND PHYSICAL EXAMINATION: A comprehensive review of the patient's medical history and the results of the most recent physical exam.

ORDERS: Medication and treatment orders made by the doctor, nurse practitioner, physician assistant, and other qualified health-care team members.

MEDICATION RECORD: Record of all medications administered by dose, date, and time.

TREATMENT RECORD: Record of all treatments received—for example, dressing changes or respiratory therapy.

PROCEDURES: Summary of diagnostic or therapeutic procedures—for example, a colonoscopy or open-heart surgery.

TESTS: Results of diagnostic evaluations, such as laboratory tests; electrocardiograms; and X-ray images or summaries of X-ray results.

PROGRESS NOTES: Regular notes on the patient's status by the interdisciplinary care team.

CONSULTATIONS: Clinical notes and recommendations from specialized diagnosticians or care providers.

CONSENTS: Permissions signed by the patient for procedures, tests, or access to the chart, as well as releases—for example, the release signed by the patient when leaving the facility against medical advice.

FLOW RECORDS: Tables or charts that track specific aspects of patient care that occur on a routine basis.

CARE PLAN: Treatment goals and plan for care within the facility or after discharge.

DISCHARGE: Final instructions for the patient and final reports by the care team before the patient leaves the hospital and the chart is closed and stored.

INSURANCE INFORMATION: Health-care-benefit coverage and hospital contact information for the insurance provider.

A hospital may subdivide or expand these general categories. For example, a psychiatric hospital may have a special section for psychometric testing, and an acute-care hospital may have sections specifically for operations, X-ray reports, or electrocardiograms. In addition, allergies, do-not-resuscitate (DNR) orders, and other significant information may be displayed prominently on large colored stickers or in special chart sections.

The information in the chart must be clear and concise so that people utilizing it can easily access what they need to know. The chart can also help in clinical problem-solving by tracking the patient's baseline statistics and status on admission, orders given and treatments provided to deal with specific problems, and the patient's responses. Another reason for clear documentation is the possibility that the record might some day be used for legal purposes—in a malpractice suit, for instance. When things go wrong, hospitals are fond of using the phrase "adverse events" to describe medical errors of all kinds, including those that cause death. In most court cases that involve patient care, chart contents are routinely cited and admitted as evidence.

Medical charts are usually managed by the nursing-station clerk while your loved one is a patient. After your loved one is discharged, the chart will be stored in the medical records department. Typically, state or provincial laws govern how long and where charts are stored.

> **ASKED AND ANSWERED:** Fearing legal repercussions, many hospitals will typically duck and run from any claims of medical error, a leading cause of hospital deaths. However, new evidence suggests that those hospitals that come clean about causing an "adverse event" often avoid expensive lawsuits and are better conditioned to prevent recurrences.

How to Make a Chart

Most hospitals have very specific guidelines for making chart entries. The following would be considered typical:

> Include date and time on all records.
> Include the patient's full name and other identifiers (i.e., medical record number, date of birth) on all records.
> Mark continued records clearly (i.e., signify if a note continues on reverse of page or on another page).
> Sign each page of documentation.
> Use blue or black non-erasable ink on handwritten records.
> Keep records in chronological order.
> Prevent disposal or obliteration of any records.
> Note any documentation errors and correct clearly by drawing one line through the error, correcting it, and then initialing the area.

Avoid excess empty space on the page.

Avoid abbreviations when possible, or use only universally accepted abbreviations.

Avoid other unclear documentation, such as illegible penmanship or unexplained punctuation points like "!" and "?."

Avoid including contradictory information. For example, if a nurse documents that a patient has complained of abdominal pain throughout the shift, while the doctor documents that the patient is free of pain, these discrepancies should be discussed and clarified.

Provide objective rather than subjective information, and do not allow personality conflicts between staff to enter into the notes. All events involving the patient should be described as objectively as possible. For instance, describe a hostile patient by simply stating the facts, such as what the patient said or did and surrounding circumstances or response of staff, without using derogatory or judgmental language.

Document any occurrence that might affect the patient, like an adverse reaction to a drug. Only documented information is considered credible in court. Undocumented information is considered questionable and is therefore open to challenge, since there is no written record of its occurrence.

Always use the current date and time with documentation. For example, if a note is added after the fact, it can be labeled "addendum" and inserted in correct chronological order instead of inserted on the date of the actual occurrence.

Record actual statements of patients or other individuals in quotes.

Never leave the chart in an unprotected environment where unauthorized individuals could read or alter the contents.

Maybe you can borrow some ideas from these guidelines as you build your own chart, taking note of the need for clarity and precision when it comes to making entries. While your loved one is still a patient, if he or she gives permission, you might be allowed to read the hospital medical chart, but you won't have a personal record of your loved one's diagnosis, prognosis, treatment, and recovery. At the back of the book is a Caregiver's Chart and Personal Journal that you can use to build and maintain your own chart. Let it evolve to parallel your loved one's official record, expanding it to become a personal as well as a clinical chronicle of the hospital stay. Enter all the responses to your questions to the staff about medications, tests, and therapies—and include your own comments and observations about your loved one's progress. Leave room to express the uncertainties and disappointments of setbacks, but also be sure to acknowledge the moments of joy that can follow welcome breakthroughs. Remember that you are part of the bumpy recovery process yourself, and use these pages to reflect on its twists and turns. By the time you've made your last entry, you will have created more than a journal of care. You will have created a unique piece of family history. That's something no hospital can ever do.

The Caregiver's Chart and Personal Journal consists of two quick-reference sheets, one for day one, which allows you to fill in some baseline information and get started, and one for subsequent days—you can make photocopies or scans for more days and fill in each day's number in the space provided (see copies nearby in this chapter, and see the tear-out sheets at the back of the book).

Medications ("Meds")

Hospital doctors can select from thousands of medications that have a specific purpose. Some are administered routinely, some of those to treat conditions that can result directly from a long stay in a hospital bed. You have a right to ask the nurse for a list of the medications administered to your loved one. Those below are among the most common. They are listed alphabetically by generic name; the most recognizable brand names, if any, are given in parentheses.

> *Acetaminophen (Tylenol)*—Prescribed to relieve mild to moderate pain and/or fever. Tylenol 3 (acetaminophen with codeine) is available only by prescription.
>
> *Acetylsalicylic acid (ASA; aspirin)*—Prescribed to relieve pain, fever, and inflammation. A blood thinner, it also reduces the ability of certain cells in the blood to clot.

Caregiver's Chart and Personal Journal
(Make as many photocopies as you need.)

Day 1   Date: _____

Patient Information

Name of Patient:

Age:

Family Doctor:

Blood Type:

Allergies:

Current Medications:

Preexisting Health Issues:

Next of Kin:

Principal Caregiver:

Designated Family Spokesperson (if different):

Important Phone Numbers for Family and Friends:

Available Dates and Times for Visiting/Care:

Hospital Information

Name of Hospital:
Address:

Date of Admission:

Reason for Admission:

Expected Length of Stay:

Actual Length of Stay:

Unit/Room Number:

Visiting Hours:

Treatment Plan:

Primary Doctor or Surgeon:

    Direct Line and/or Pager Number:

Unit Charge Nurse:

    Direct Line and/or Pager Number:

Nursing Station Direct Line:

Support Services Names and Contact Numbers:

Dietitian:

Pharmacist:

Physical Therapist (Physiotherapist):

Occupational Therapist:

Social Worker:

Chaplain:

Discharge Planner:

Discharge Plan

Acceptable (yes/no):

Issues to Be Discussed:

Tests Performed (blood work, X-rays, MRIs, CT [CAT] scans, etc.)

In Room:

Out of Room:

Results:

Procedures Performed (line installation, intubation, dressing changes, etc.):

Patient's Reaction:

Medications Administered:

Patient's Reaction:

Attending Doctor's Assessment:

Specialist Assessment (if applicable):

Dietary Changes:

Therapy—Physical and Occupational:

Therapy—Other (speech, etc.):

Grooming Tasks:

Assigned to:

Bedside Assistance Provided by Caregiver:

Patient's Mood and Behavior:

Issues Raised with Care Staff:

Outcome of Discussion:

Notes/Comments/Observations:

Caregiver's Chart and Personal Journal
(Make as many photocopies as you need.)

Day no. _____   Date: _____

Tests Performed (blood work, X-rays, MRIs, CT scans, etc.)

    In Room:

    Out of Room:

Results:

Procedures Performed (line installation, intubation, dressing changes, etc.):

    Patient's Reaction:

Medications Administered:

    Patient's Reaction:

Attending Doctor's Assessment:

Specialist Assessment (if applicable):

Dietary Changes:

Therapy—Physical and Occupational:

Therapy—Other (speech, etc.):

Grooming Tasks:

Assigned to:

Bedside Assistance Provided by Caregiver:

Patient's Mood and Behavior:

Issues Raised with Care Staff:

Outcome of Discussion:

Notes/Comments/Observations:

Adenosine (Adenocard) injection—Specified when the heart is functioning improperly in order to kick-start it.

Amiodarone (Codarone)—Specified when the heart has irregular rhythm (arrhythmia) in order to bring it back to a regular rhythm. Usually continued in a monitored environment until the arrhythmia is adequately controlled.

Amlodipine (Norvasc)—Prescribed to treat mild to moderate hypertension (high blood pressure). Eases ongoing chest pain caused by angina.

Antibiotics, including amoxicillin (Amoxil), clarithromycin (Biaxin), erythromycin (E-Mycin), azithromycin (Zithromax), cefazolin (Ancef), and cefotaxime (Claforan)—Prescribed to treat and prevent bacterial infections.

Antifungals, including ketoconazole (Nizoral) and fluconazole (Diflucan)—Prescribed to treat and prevent fungal infections.

Aspirin.—See acetylsalicylic acid

Atropine—Used during cardiopulmonary resuscitation (CPR). Increases heart rate and blood pressure.

Benzodiazepines, including diazepam (Valium), lorazepam (Ativan), alprazolam (Xanax), midazolam (Versed), clonazepam (Rivotril)—Prescribed to treat anxiety, insomnia, panic disorders, seizures, and muscle spasms and to help presurgery patients relax. Each drug in this class has a specific purpose or set of purposes, and results may vary between patients. Administering these drugs can be a trial-and-error process. Sometimes a doctor may change a drug after observing the patient's response—an appropriate action when results are not as expected.

Budesonide (Pulmicort), an inhaled steroid medication—Prescribed to treat inflammation of the airways, such as in bronchial asthma.

Calcium gluconate injection—Prescribed to replenish calcium levels quickly. Also used in the treatment of black widow spider bites to relieve cramping.

Clopidogrel (Plavix)—Prescribed to help prevent strokes or heart attacks by halting the formation of dangerous blood clots.

Corticosteroids, including prednisone and dexamethasone (Decadron)—Used to treat a large variety of conditions, from brain tumors to skin conditions. Can help control stress response and immune response and regulate inflammation, carbohydrate metabolism, protein catabolism, blood electrolyte levels, and behavior.

Dextrose, a form of sugar—Commonly injected to raise blood sugar to normal levels.

Digoxin (Lanoxin)—Used to treat mild to moderate heart failure. Normally continued after the condition is under control to help prevent recurrence.

Docusate sodium (Colace)—Used to soften the stool and prevent painful passage.

Dopamine—Prescribed to increase heart rate and blood pressure in patients suffering from shock, which it does by acting on the sympathetic nervous system (source of the stressed fight-or-flight response).

Epinephrine (EpiPen)—Injected to treat life-threatening allergic reactions caused by insect bites, foods, medications, latex, and other things. People allergic to peanuts are encouraged to carry a shot of epinephrine at all times because untreated symptoms can swiftly lead to death. Also used to restart the heart when other methods have failed and to prolong the effects of intraspinal and local anesthetics.

Furosemide (Lasix)—Used to treat edema (excess fluid) associated with congestive heart failure, cirrhosis of the liver, and kidney disease. Also used to treat mild to moderate hypertension (high blood pressure).

Heparin—Used as a blood thinner in the treatment of thrombosis (blood clot) and also to prevent clotting during dialysis. Could also be used with high-risk patients undergoing certain kinds of surgery.

Hyoscine, scopolamine, butylbromide (Buscopan) — Prescribed to relieve stomach cramps.

Ibuprofen (Advil) — Prescribed for the temporary relief of pain and fever. Used alternately with acetaminophen and acetylsalicylic acid (ASA; aspirin), depending on variables in each patient's condition.

Insulin — Prescribed to lower and regulate blood sugar levels in diabetic patients.

Lidocaine (Xylocaine) — Used as a topical anesthetic to relieve itching, burning, and pain from skin inflammations; sometimes applied before minor surgery, causing a "freezing" effect. Injected to help regulate heart rhythm.

Lorazepam (Ativan) — Used for short-term relief of anxiety. Sometimes administered in advance of surgery.

Magnesium carbonate (Gaviscon) — An antacid prescribed to relieve heartburn and gastroesophageal reflux disease (GERD).

Magnesium citrate (Citroma) — Used to stimulate and clean out the bowels as a preparation for various procedures, including barium enemas and bowel surgery. Functions best on an empty stomach.

Mannitol — Prescribed to prevent or treat excess body water in certain kidney conditions. Has also been used to reduce brain swelling that results from head injuries, but this use of the drug remains controversial, with some researchers arguing that it can worsen the condition.

Metoprolol succinate (Betaloc), a beta-blocker — Used to treat hypertension (high blood pressure) and angina (chest pain), to correct irregular heartbeat, to prevent migraine headache, and to treat tremors. Often administered during heart attacks to reduce the stress on the heart and to reduce any damage that occurs.

Naloxone (Narcan) — Prescribed to prevent or reverse the effects of opioids (morphine, etc.). Acts quickly. Often used in cases of drug overdose.

Nitroglycerin (Nitro-Dur) — Used to treat conditions like angina (chest pain) and possibly prevent heart attacks by widening the arteries, which allows more blood to flow through them to critical areas of the heart.

Opioids, including morphine, codeine, fentanyl, methadone, oxycodone + acetaminophen (Percocet), oxycodone + acetylsalicylic acid (Percodan), hydrocodone + acetaminophen (Vicodin)—Prescribed to treat chronic or acute pain associated with surgical or medical conditions like trauma, heart failure, and terminal cancer. Most opioids are potentially addictive (or at least habit-forming) and are therefore administered or prescribed according to very stringent guidelines.

Phenytoin (Dilantin)—Prescribed to control seizures and to prevent and treat seizures that might occur during or following neurosurgery.

Propofol (Diprivan)—Used as a short-acting general anesthetic and used to sedate patients undergoing diagnostic procedures. Also used to sedate patients receiving oxygen in intensive-care units.

Ringer's lactate, lactated Ringer's solution—Used for fluid restoration after a blood loss due to trauma, surgery, or a burn injury. Also used to induce urination in patients with kidney failure.

Salbutamol (Ventolin)—Inhaled or introduced down the bronchial tube; used to help relieve spasms within the lungs such as those associated with asthma and chronic bronchitis. Also used to prevent exercise-induced asthma.

Sodium bicarbonate—Used to bring the pH balance of the body back to normal, typically resulting in less acidic blood or urine.

Sodium polystyrene (Kayexalate)—Used to treat hyperkalemia (an abnormally high concentration of potassium in the blood) by removing excess potassium.

Tenecteplase (TNKase)—Administered through an IV line shortly after the occurrence of an acute heart attack, it acts as a quick clot-buster when timing is critical, but serious risks include bleeding and, in elderly patients, the possibility of a stroke.

Once you know what medications your loved one is taking, you will want to ask the nurse about them. Ask these questions about all the medications being prescribed.

> What is it for?
>
> How often is it given?
>
> What are the side effects, and what should I do if my loved one develops side effects?
>
> Are there any foods, drinks, or activities that my loved one should avoid while on the medication?
>
> Will my loved one be on this medication at home?
>
> Is it safe to take this medication with other medications or supplements?

SMART MOVES: **Medication Alert**

- Make sure nursing staff are fully aware of any over-the-counter medications, herbal remedies, and alternative therapies (such as acupuncture) that your loved one may be currently using or may have recently used.

- Alert the charge nurse to your loved one's allergies or adverse reactions to medications, dye, iodine, shellfish, radiology contrast materials, anesthetics—and anything else.

- Ask about any medications your loved one is taking.

Lab Tests

Most hospital patients endure a regular round of regular lab tests, many requiring the drawing of blood samples and all of them ordered to assist with diagnosis as well as treatment. Here are some examples common to most patients, no matter what their illness or disorder.

Arterial Blood Gas (ABG)

Purpose: To test the blood for an imbalance in oxygen and carbon dioxide levels.

Note: Normally administered when breathing is difficult or when a patient is hyperventilating. The result could help determine the cause, which may be a metabolic or kidney disorder. May also be used to monitor ongoing oxygen therapy for respiratory patients, and may also be used during certain surgeries.

Blood Cultures

Purpose: To test for bacteria in the blood.

Note: Bloodstream infections (known as sepsis or septicemia) typically migrate from another part of the body to the bloodstream. They can be life-threatening and require urgent treatment. Symptoms include chills, fever, nausea, rapid heartbeat, confusion, and decreased urine output. Infants, the elderly, surgical patients, and people receiving immunosuppressive therapy can be especially vulnerable.

Blood Sugar or Glucose Test

Purpose: To check the level of sugar in the blood.

Note: The normal level is 100 milligrams per deciliter (mg/dl). If the level is higher than 100 but less than 199, a pre-diabetic condition may be indicated. Fasting is recommended before the test. Sometimes a random urine sample is used instead of blood.

Blood Urea Nitrogen (BUN) Test

Purpose: To determine how well the kidneys are working.

Note: Can also be used to evaluate a person's general health. Frequently administered to emergency patients who arrive with acute illnesses. Increased BUN levels suggest that kidney function is impaired.

Cardiac Enzyme Test

Purpose: To check for injury to the heart resulting in a blockage of blood flow.

Note: When any part of the heart muscle has been injured, it releases certain chemicals, which this blood test identifies and measures.

Complete Blood Count (CBC)

Purpose: To check the levels of different cells in the blood.

Note: Actually a comprehensive panel of tests rather than a single test, the CBC is routinely administered to most hospital patients in order to screen, help diagnose, or monitor a large variety of conditions. The tests provide quite a bit of information.

White blood cell (WBC) count—A calculation of the number of white blood cells per volume of blood. Both increases and decreases can be significant.

White blood cell differential—A classification of the types of white blood cells present. There are five different types of white blood cells, each with its own function in protecting the body from infection.

Red blood cell (RBC) count—A calculation of the number of red blood cells per volume of blood. Both increases and decreases can point to abnormal conditions.

Hemoglobin test—A measurement of the amount of oxygen-carrying protein in the blood.

Hematocrit—A measurement of the amount of space that red blood cells take up in the blood. It is reported as a percentage.

Platelet count—A calculation of the number of platelets in a given volume of blood. Both increases and decreases can point to abnormal conditions, such as excess bleeding or clotting problems.

Mean platelet volume (MPV)—A measurement of the average size of the platelets. New platelets are larger than old ones, and an increased MPV occurs when increased numbers of platelets are being produced. An MPV gives a doctor information about platelet production in the bone marrow.

Mean corpuscular volume (MCV)—A measurement of the average size of the red blood cells. The MCV is elevated when the red blood cells are larger than normal (macrocytic), as in anemia caused by a vitamin B12 deficiency. When the MCV is decreased, the red blood cells are smaller than normal (microcytic), as is often seen in iron deficiency anemia.

Mean corpuscular hemoglobin (MCH)—A calculation of the amount of oxygen-carrying hemoglobin inside the red blood cells. Since macrocytic red blood cells are larger than either normal or microcytic red blood cells, they also tend to have higher MCH values.

Mean corpuscular hemoglobin concentration (MCHC)—A calculation of the concentration of hemoglobin inside the red blood cells. Decreased MCHC values (hypochromia) are seen when the hemoglobin is abnormally diluted inside the red cells, as in iron deficiency anemia and in thalassemia (an inherited blood disease). Increased MCHC values (hyperchromia) are seen when the hemoglobin is abnormally concentrated inside the red cells, as in hereditary spherocytosis (a rare congenital disorder).

Red cell distribution width (RDW)—A calculation of the variation in the size of the red blood cells. In some anemias, such as pernicious anemia, the amount of variation (anisocytosis) in their size (along with variation in shape, or poikilocytosis) causes an increase in the RDW.

Coagulation (PT/INR)

Purpose: To determine how long it takes for blood to clot.

Note: PT (prothrombin time) and INR (international normalized ratio), both measures of blood-clotting time, are often used to monitor the effectiveness of blood-thinning drugs such as warfarin. They are also used in conjunction with PTT (activated partial thromboplastin time) and are often administered for surgical prescreening.

Creatine Kinase (CK) Test

Purpose: To determine if a heart attack has occurred or if other muscles in the body have been damaged.

Note: When any muscle is injured (including the heart), it releases a specific chemical into the blood, which this test looks for.

Creatinine Test

Purpose: To assess kidney function.

Note: May be ordered along with the BUN test when the patient has a known kidney disorder or a disease that might affect kidney function or when a CT scan is planned.

Cross and Type Test

Purpose: To identify and cross-match blood type.

Note: Typically administered on admission to a hospital if the patient's blood type is unknown or in doubt, the test is necessary in case a blood transfusion is required, particularly for surgery patients. There are eight different blood types, so compatibility and matching are important. But in an emergency, anyone can receive type O blood (the most common in North America), which is why people with type O blood (particularly O negative) are called universal donors.

D-Dimer Test

Purpose: To test for thrombosis (blood clot).

Note: Typically ordered when a patient reports leg pain, swelling, discoloration, tenderness, or edema. Introduced in the 1990s, it is a quick and noninvasive way to rule out excess or abnormal blood clotting.

Drug Screen

Purpose: To check for drugs and medications present in the system, ingested either on purpose or by accident.

Note: Often indicated in cases of suspected drug abuse but also useful to determine whether a patient's medications are compatible with each other—or whether something like alcohol is causing unwanted side effects.

Electrolyte Test

Purpose: To detect from a blood sample any problem with the body's electrolyte balance.

Note: Electrolytes are essential to help regulate the heart, the nervous system, fluid balance, and oxygen delivery, among other things. A common cause of electrolyte disturbance is renal failure. People with bulimia or anorexia are at especially high risk.

Lactic Acid Test

Purpose: To determine whether blood cells have enough oxygen and to check the body's acid-base balance.

Note: Lactate (the electrically charged form of lactic acid) is usually present in low levels in the blood and contributes to a person's energy. Increased levels can lead to muscular weakness, rapid breathing, nausea, sweating, and even coma. Unless the test is given under emergency conditions, patients are expected to fast for eight to ten hours beforehand.

Liver Function Test

Purpose: To determine how efficiently the liver is working.

Note: The most obvious symptom of a liver problem is jaundice; other symptoms are dark urine, unusual weight change, vomiting, diarrhea, chronic fatigue, and vomiting of blood. The test is a panel of many different tests run from a blood sample. Among them are tests for the following.

Alanine aminotransferase (ALT)—An enzyme mainly found in the liver. Testing for it is the best way to detect hepatitis.

Alkaline phosphatase (ALP)—An enzyme related to the bile ducts, often increased when the ducts are blocked.

Aspartate aminotransferase (AST)—An enzyme found in the liver and a few other places, particularly the heart and other muscles in the body.

Bilirubin—A reddish-yellow bile pigment. Two different tests of bilirubin are often used together, especially if a person has jaundice: a total bilirubin test measures all the bilirubin in the blood, and a direct bilirubin test measures a form of bilirubin that is conjugated (combined with another compound) in the liver.

Albumin—The main protein made by the liver. The albumin test tells whether the liver is making an adequate amount of this protein. A total protein test measures albumin and all other proteins in the blood, including antibodies made to help fight off infections.

Methicillin-Resistant *Staphylococcus aureus* (MRSA) Swabs

Purpose: To check for bacteria resistant to regular antibiotics.

Note: An MRSA infection, colloquially called a superbug, is dangerous because it can spread rapidly to other patients. A swab is taken at the site of the infection (a wound or a lesion), and the resulting culture is analyzed and identified in the lab before treatment is determined. An MRSA infection, a condition traditionally associated with a hospital, is now starting to appear anywhere people are in close, constant contact—for example, the locker rooms of sports teams.

Osmolality Test

Purpose: To determine the fluid balance in the body.

Note: A sample is drawn from either the blood or urine. Used to help evaluate the body's water balance and its ability to produce and concentrate urine; to detect the presence of toxins like methanol (wood alcohol) or ethylene glycol (antifreeze); and to help monitor medications that might affect fluid balance. Typically ordered when a patient has such symptoms as excessive thirst, nausea, headache, lethargy, and seizures or is in a coma that may have been caused by ingesting methanol or ethylene glycol.

Throat Swabs

Purpose: To determine the cause of a sore throat.

Note: Ordered if a bacterial respiratory infection is suspected. A sample for lab analysis is taken by swabbing the back of the throat. The most typical bacterial respiratory infection is a group A streptococcal infection. "Strep throat" is somewhat common among hospital patients but is easily treated with antibiotics.

Troponin

Purpose: To determine from a blood sample if a heart attack has occurred.

Note: Often administered to people who report to the emergency department complaining of prolonged chest pains, this test checks for the presence of a chemical released when there has been a heart attack or damage to the heart. It is usually combined with other heart tests when the symptoms continue and is administered several times during a twelve-to-sixteen-hour period as part of ongoing monitoring.

Urinalysis

Purpose: To screen and diagnose potential kidney and metabolic disorders.

Note: Often administered upon hospital admission. A urine sample can be useful to assess a variety of conditions, including a possible urinary tract infection. Urinalysis is particularly indicated for emergency patients reporting abdominal or back pain, painful or frequent urination, or blood in the urine. The results can also raise a red flag that something may be wrong elsewhere in the body.

SMART MOVES: **Bedside Vigilance**

- Discourage your loved one from trying to get out of bed without help unless he or she is fully ambulatory. Bed rails, IV lines, and other hospital equipment may get in the way, and your loved one may get hurt or fall. Suggest that your loved one always ask for assistance if you are not available to help.

- Use the call bell for any needs. Don't wait until the last minute to call for help, because the nurse may be tending other patients and could take time to respond.

- Be aware that your loved one should be turned every two hours to prevent bedsores. Ask the nurse for help if needed, and be ready to offer your own assistance, but be sure your loved one never stays in the same position for more than two hours. You might ask the nurse to show you the best way to turn the patient yourself.

- With the kindest of intentions, visitors may bring food for your loved one, figuring that a change from the hospital diet would be welcome. Accept it—but if you have concerns, check with the nurse before giving it to your loved one in case the food might conflict with any dietary restrictions or medications.

Emergency Codes

When you sit quietly by the bed while your loved one is enjoying a rare chance to doze, there may be times when your attention drifts to what you hear from the hospital public address speakers overhead. Mostly you will hear pages for staff, announcements of events, and notifications to visitors that visiting hours are over—the routine daily business of any hospital. But sometimes code calls are broadcast throughout the hospital to alert staff to emergency situations. The emergencies are color-coded; each type of emergency is assigned a color. Most people who watch medical dramas on television already know what a Code Blue call is, but the rest of the emergency color palette may not be familiar.

Code calls, which are typically announced very clearly and calmly three times in succession, always include the hospital location of the emergency. A later announcement may confirm that the emergency has been resolved.

What should you do if you hear a code call? Nothing. Wait for further instructions; if any are forthcoming, they will be broadcast throughout the hospital. An example would be a call for evacuation. The exception to doing nothing is with a Code Blue call. If you hear that and are in a hallway, get ready to step quickly aside. Otherwise you may be run over by a crash cart, a mobile clinical toolkit packed with all the devices and medications required to save someone's life. It will be pushed or dragged along by several health-care providers in a hurry.

Bear in mind that different countries have different codes. In North America, there can even be variations from hospital to hospital and state to state or province to province. To avoid confusion and panic among patients and visitors, most hospitals will post an explanation of their code colors in prominent places like elevators and notice boards.

These are the most common codes in use in the United States:

Code Red	Fire
Code Blue	Adult medical emergency
Code White	Pediatric medical emergency
Code Gray	Combative person with no weapon
Code Silver	Combative person with a weapon and/or a hostage situation
Code Pink	Infant abduction
Code Purple	Child abduction
Code Yellow	Bomb threat
Code Orange	Hazardous materials spill or release
Code Triage Internal	An internal disaster
Code Triage External	An external disaster

And these are the most common codes in use in Canada:

Code Red	Fire
Code Blue	Cardiac arrest
Code Green	Evacuation
Code White	Violent person
Code Yellow	Missing patient
Code Orange	External disaster
Code Brown	Hazardous spill
Code Purple	Emergency department can no longer accept patients; divert to other hospitals
Code Black	Bomb threat
Code Gray	Internal disaster

If you happen to hear a code call while you're in the hospital, consider recording it with the date and time in your own Caregiver's Chart and Personal Journal. Why not? It's part of your hospital experience, one more reminder that you are now in a place where emergencies don't punch a time clock.

8
Recovery (III)
Partnering with the Care Team and
Planning for Home

Hospital patients may yearn for undisturbed rest during the day, but few get to enjoy it. There's always something going on—visitors who show up unexpectedly, the hum and wheeze of bedside monitoring equipment, conversations and laughter from the hallway, the muttered opinions of doctors as they bounce from room to room. And then there are the routine nursing tasks and tests, all performed by conscientious professionals who descend on patients in accordance with some mysterious schedule not shared with the people in bed.

Sometimes your loved one will leave the hospital room for a test or procedure, but many tasks, including some tests and procedures, are done right in the room. For any test or procedure, stay informed by asking the nurse the following questions:

> What is the test or procedure?
> What is it for, and why is it necessary?
> How long will it take?
> Are there any risks involved?
> (If your loved one is leaving the room) May I come along?

The Daily Routine

As your loved one's care partner, look for ways to integrate yourself into active bedside care. The routine daily nursing tasks will vary from patient to patient, but opportunities to help are indicated in the following list.

Bathing and Grooming the Patient and Providing Oral Care

Not a priority for all nurses in all settings, given heavy clinical schedules and staff shortages.

Care-partnership opportunity: You can undertake to perform regular grooming and oral care: comb your loved one's hair, soak dentures, brush and floss teeth, help with nose blowing and nail clipping, do anything else that might make your loved one both more comfortable and happier to receive other visitors.

Taking Blood Samples

To take a blood sample, a nurse inserts a needle into a vein, usually in the forearm. The drawn sample is sent to the hospital lab for analysis. The frequency of blood tests will depend on the patient's condition. Some patients may require specific blood tests several times a day.

Care-partnership opportunity: Your loved one may be squeamish about needles. Drawing a blood sample is usually a quick process, and you may be able to distract your loved one by a brief reference to the weather or an impending visit by a family member.

Monitoring Blood Pressure

At most hospitals the bedside staff use an upper-arm cuff and a hand inflation bulb with a pressure control valve to apply pressure—and a stethoscope to listen for certain sounds. The ideal blood pressure for an adult when the heart is at rest, all other things being equal, is 120/80 (pronounced "one twenty over eighty").

Care-partnership opportunity: By reassuring your loved one that there will be no discomfort, you can help ease any apparent anxiety that might elevate blood pressure and affect the result of the blood pressure test.

Monitoring Breath Sounds

A stethoscope is placed on the chest to listen to the patient breathing—a simple way to assess lung function.

Care-partnership opportunity: Make sure the person with the stethoscope briefly rubs the end of it to warm it before placing it on the skin. Encourage your loved one to breathe normally.

Caring for the Catheter

Maintenance of the bladder catheter, if there is one, requires draining the urine collection bag, cleaning the catheter entry area, and confirming that the collection bag remains below the bladder so that gravity assures that the urine will flow out (rather than the reverse).

Care-partnership opportunity: Emphasize to your loved one that this is a routine procedure and that there is no cause for alarm. Make sure the collection bag remains below your loved one—it is typically attached to the bed on the rail below the mattress and can sometimes be knocked out of position.

Changing Intravenous Sites

The sites don't need to be changed every day. The task is usually performed according to a schedule. Not changing IV sites could lead to infection at the entry site after a period of time.

Care-partnership opportunity: You can stand by in case your loved one becomes apprehensive or physically uncomfortable during the procedure and be ready to offer comfort and reassurance.

Changing Dressings

Depending on the severity of the wound, a dressing may have several layers of absorbent material that need to be periodically removed, and the wound may need to be cleansed and then repacked with sterile gauze or bandages to reduce the risk of an infection that might interfere with the healing process.

Care-partnership opportunity: You can remain at the nurse's side and offer to hand over fresh dressings or supplies as needed. Watch carefully what happens, in case you need to change a dressing after your loved one has been discharged.

Giving an Enema

To give an enema, a quantity of fluid is infused into the rectum through a tube inserted into the anus to help induce a bowel movement.

Care-partnership opportunity: Receiving an enema is not usually painful, but it certainly can be unpleasant, and many patients find it humiliating. You can help by assuring that your loved one's personal privacy and dignity are respected, even by simply repositioning the sheet so that it discreetly covers the area.

Flushing the Intravenous Line

Forcing a quantity of fluid (usually sterile saltwater) through the IV line clears the line and displaces its contents into the body quickly.

Care-partnership opportunity: Be sure your loved one understands that this is a routine procedure. And if you were in conversation before the nurse arrived, carry on chatting throughout.

Applying the Glasgow Coma Scale

A neurological test, the Glasgow Coma Scale was invented in 1974 by two University of Glasgow professors to assess a person's level of consciousness. The test giver attempts to elicit reactions (eye, voice, move-

ment, etc.) and rates them according to the scale. Comas are rated as severe, moderate, or minor.

Care-partnership opportunity: Based on your personal knowledge
of the patient, you can help confirm normal as well as unusual responses to various stimuli.

Making a Head-to-Toe Assessment

This assessment, a quick but thorough check of a person, including a
basic check of inner parts of the body (such as breath sounds and bowel
sounds), is performed using only a stethoscope and is not intended to
substitute for tests like X-rays and CT scans.

Care-partnership opportunity: You can provide any health history
or lifestyle information that might augment the assessment.

Inserting an IV Line

This sterile procedure involves inserting a needle covered by a tiny,
flexible "straw" into a vein. The needle is attached to a flexible tube
(line) with fluid in it that typically leads to a bag hanging from a nearby
pole. Once the needle is inserted, the fluid in the bag—which may be
anything from blood to medication—can flow into the patient's bloodstream.

Care-partnership opportunity: Watch for any seepage, including
blood, around the entry point. Notify the nurse immediately if you suspect the line may have become detached, crimped or blocked.

Intubating the Patient

When a patient cannot breathe adequately on his or her own, a tube is
inserted through the mouth into the airway, and a ventilator (respirator)
supplies oxygen through the tube. The supply can be adjusted according to the patient's need.

Care-partnership opportunity: The normal human reflex is to gag
and reject anything that's being inserted down the throat, and nurses

are trained to overcome resistance by using moderate force when required. You can support your loved one as she or he endures this sometimes uncomfortable procedure by explaining its necessity and by holding a hand throughout.

Collecting Spinal Fluid with a Lumbar Puncture

This sterile procedure is normally performed using a local anesthetic to prevent it from being unnecessarily painful. Ideally, the patient lies on his or her side, curled up with the knees hugged to the chest in order to maximize the space between the bones in the lower back. To reduce risk, the patient must stay completely still while a hollow needle is inserted into the space between specific bones. The collected spinal fluid is sent to the lab for diagnostic purposes.

Care-partnership opportunity: You can calm your loved one and encourage absolute immobility through a procedure that frequently causes anxiety and discomfort.

Administering Medications

Nurses administer regular doses of the medications ordered for each patient according to a schedule that seldom varies. Most patients receive medications several times a day.

Care-partnership opportunity: You can report physical or emotional reactions that might indicate a need to review and/or change medications.

Giving a Mini Mental Status Exam

This exam, sometimes called the Folstein test, is a list of thirty simple questions given to quickly assess cognitive function. The questions sample arithmetic, memory, and orientation skills. Examples: "What is today's date?" and "Can you tell me where you are?" Any score above twenty-four is considered normal. A score below twenty might indicate dementia.

Care-partnership opportunity: You can assist with orientation questions by simply being a reassuring presence and possibly easing distress and confusion if the patient starts to get frustrated attempting to respond.

Helping with Mobilization

Time (typically up to thirty minutes) spent sitting upright in a nearby comfortable chair will often have cardiovascular benefits for patients confined to bed for long periods. But monitoring for signs of breathing instability or discomfort is important.

Care-partnership opportunity: You can relieve a nurse of the need to remain with your loved one if you undertake to monitor responses and immediately alert staff to any evidence of physical or emotional distress.

Applying a Neuro/Stroke Assessment Scale

Various scales are designed to assess nerve function in conscious stroke patients, but they are also useful in assessing other conditions. The scales are typically used to assess level of consciousness, orientation, aphasia (loss of the ability to understand language), and motor strength. Each condition is rated.

Care-partnership opportunity: By carefully explaining what is happening and why, you can help the patient relax through a test procedure that can sometimes be challenging and therefore stressful. Make certain your loved one understands that any discouraging results could be only temporary—they should not be taken as final.

Giving Nutrition Intravenously

Patients who cannot (or should not) take food orally receive their nutrition in liquid form, delivered intravenously from a bag suspended from a nearby pole. The procedure, called total parenteral nutrition (TPN), provides essential calories, protein, and fat to the patient.

Care-partnership opportunity: You can help monitor the level in the bag to confirm that it is emptying at a steady rate, check for steady flow by examining the line, and alert staff if the bag is empty and might need replacement.

Assessing Peak Expiratory Flow

The patient undergoing this basic procedure to check lung capacity and performance is asked to inhale deeply, wrap the lips around the tube of the testing instrument, and exhale forcefully.

Care-partnership opportunity: You can act as a personal cheerleader and encourage the patient to exhale as forcefully as possible. Be sensitive to the possibility that it may take extraordinary effort.

Assessing Pupil Size

This quick test amounts to estimating the size of a patient's pupils (the black part of the eye). Larger or smaller variances from normal pupil size can have diagnostic significance.

Care-partnership opportunity: Reassure your loved one that this is a very brief but important test and that full cooperation requires only minimal effort.

Checking Pupil Reactivity

This check to determine whether a patient's pupils react to light is done by first darkening the hospital room and then shining a light directly into first one eye and then the other. Normally, the pupil shrinks in the light, but if there is no change, the nerve controlling this function could be impaired.

Care-partnership opportunity: Darkening the room suddenly can confuse some patients. Assure your loved one that normal room light will be restored very quickly after this brief test.

Giving a Rectal Exam

To give a rectal exam a lubricated finger is inserted into the rectum to check for rectal tone and confirm that the nerves still have control over the area.

Care-partnership opportunity: A rectal exam can be embarrassing for any patient, but you can help by being as offhand and as casual as you can about the procedure while assuring that the patient's privacy and dignity are maintained.

Repositioning the Patient

Patients who are unable to move themselves are shifted in the bed (ideally, every two hours) to relieve pressure on the bony parts of the body that rest against the mattress. Repositioning is usually performed to inhibit the development of painful bedsores, a preventable condition that occurs too frequently in hospitals.

Care-partnership opportunity: You can help to move your loved one and make sure this is done frequently. Be sure to learn how best to move the patient.

Caring for the Stoma

Cleaning and caring for the area of skin where a patient's colostomy bag is attached is necessary to keep the skin healthy.

Care-partnership opportunity: Be alert to any sign of inflammation or discharge around the site. That could be a sign of possible infection, and you should notify the nurse immediately.

Monitoring Urine Output

Maintaining a record of the amount of urine produced over time (usually twenty-four hours) is necessary to assess kidney function. It is also useful to make sure the body is not being overloaded by fluid (by mouth or intravenous line). Fluid intake should not be significantly more than the kidneys are able to produce as urine.

Care-partnership opportunity: Watch for signs of excessive thirst in your loved one, allowing for the dry warm air that's characteristic of most hospitals, and alert the staff if anything appears to be abnormal, such as frequent requests for water. You want to help assure that the kidneys are not overtaxed.

Assessing Vital Signs

This appraisal of the basic body functions, including heart rate, blood pressure, respiration, and temperature, can be performed manually, or it can be performed automatically and constantly by machine.

Care-partnership opportunity: It's an important status checker, and if it's performed manually, you can explain the purpose of this routine appraisal to your loved one by emphasizing its very useful role in basic daily care.

Taking an X-Ray

X-rays can be taken with a portable machine. To do this, an X-ray technician places a special plate under or behind the patient, wheels the machine over to the bedside, and clears the immediate vicinity for a quick exposure that lasts only a few seconds.

Care-partnership opportunity: You can help shift and settle your loved one comfortably into the optimal position required by the X-ray technician, who is typically in a hurry to get to the next patient on the list.

SMART MOVES: **Test Time**

- Ask your loved one if he or she is comfortable with your presence at each in-room test and procedure as it comes along. If the nurse accepts your offer of assistance, make sure that's okay with your loved one. Accord your loved one the same respect for personal privacy as the staff do.

- Be aware that some nurses may politely refuse your offer of help. Try not to take it personally. They are often so focused on a task that they can't tolerate any distraction—and they are often extremely busy.

- Use the word *we* strategically in conversations with staff about your loved one's care, and make sure that nurses understand the purpose of your presence—that you are not there to be vigilant or intrusive but to provide what comfort and assistance you can.

- Watch your loved one for signs of institutionalization, a condition in which longer-stay patients become listless, unfocused, and unusually passive or compliant. It is an understandable survival response, but it can impede recovery.

- Make sure your loved one has all the help she or he needs when being transferred from the bed to a gurney or wheelchair for transport to any out-of-room test or procedure site. If your loved one has undergone the procedure before and has had problems or discomfort in the past, be sure to let the nurse know.

- Ask about the results of the test or procedure and what they mean.

Microbes: The Enemy Within

After drug companies began mass-producing penicillin in 1943, it seemed that the wonder drug could kill every nasty bug in its path. As time passed, new antibiotics were added to the medical arsenal, and the drug industry was confident that it had all of the world's known infections on the run. Development of fresh antibiotics stalled. By the late 1960s a new generation of microbes emerged that proved stubbornly resistant to penicillin and other antibiotics. The so-called superbugs were here. Since 1990 they have managed to invade the very places where infection is supposed to stop at the door: hospitals.

It has been estimated that three million North Americans pick up infections every year while they're in hospitals being treated for something else, and nearly one hundred thousand die as a direct or indirect result. Most of those deaths could be prevented if all staff and visitors washed their hands.

Since the SARS (severe acute respiratory syndrome) outbreak that hit Toronto in March 2003, hand sanitizers have become common in hospitals and other public buildings across North America. Many visitors now use them automatically on entering the hospital and again before entering the patient's room because extensive educational programs have convinced them that hands are proven carriers of bacteria.

ASKED AND ANSWERED: Although it is now widely accepted that handwashing can greatly reduce dangerous hospital infection rates, health-care providers seem slow to adapt. A 2008 study by Ontario's auditor general concluded that just 28 percent of provincial doctors wash their hands between patients, the lowest rate among that jurisdiction's care providers. To encourage daily compliance with hygiene standards, one large Toronto hospital randomly dispenses snack-sized doughnuts to staff spotted washing their hands.

Microbes breed in hospitals, easily infecting people weakened by illness. You should be aware of the most dangerous bugs, including the following.

Methicillin-Resistant *Staphylococcus aureus* (MRSA)

MRSA is a common strain of bacteria that have become resistant to certain antibiotics. Although this strain is often found on the skin and in the noses of healthy people, it is usually harmless and rarely causes infection in healthy people. It is most often seen in hospitals, where it can cause infection if it invades the body through a cut or during surgery. The infection can also develop in an open wound, such as a bedsore, or at a stoma, the site where a urinary catheter or other tube enters the body. People with long-term illnesses and people who have compromised immune systems are at increased risk of infection.

MRSA is usually transmitted to patients through people's hands, especially the hands of health-care workers contaminated with MRSA bacteria through contact with infected or colonized patients. The easiest way to prevent transmission is by washing the hands with soap and water or by using an alcohol-based hand sanitizer.

When penicillin was first used, it was highly effective against *Staphylococcus aureus* infections, but most strains of the bacteria are now resistant to the antibiotic. Now MRSA infections are treated with an antibiotic called vancomycin, which is derived from soil bacteria found in India and Indonesia. Vancomycin is extremely irritating to human tissue, so it is used only as a last resort. Still, some bacteria have become resistant even to this antibiotic—examples are the vancomycin-resistant *Staphylococcus aureus* (VRSA) and the more common vancomycin-resistant *Enterococcus* (VRE).

A hospital patient who develops an MRSA infection can expect his or her hospital stay to triple in length.

While MRSA outbreaks are fairly common in North America, some European countries, including the Netherlands, Finland, and Sweden have been aggressive in dealing with the bacteria. The Netherlands has adopted a search-and-destroy campaign—you are considered infected until tests prove that you are not. Infected people are placed in isolation, and hand-washing orders are enforced. Rates of infection have dropped dramatically, even while they've remained high in neighboring countries.

Vancomycin-Resistant *Enterococcus* (VRE)

Two species of *Enterococcus* commonly live in the intestines, but they are usually benign. *Enterococcus* infections can occur in the urinary tract, in the blood, and in wounds, including surgical wounds. Although these infections can usually be treated with antibiotics like ampicillin and vancomycin, a strain of bacteria that are resistant to both was discovered in France in 1986. Similar strains can now be found all over the world.

VRE is thought to be passed to people through contact with animals or by eating meat. Once the meat is eaten, the bacteria sit dormant in the person's gut until they come into contact with an antibiotic. At that point the VRE can spread to the rest of the body. And since many patients in hospitals are put on some kind of antibiotic therapy during the course of their treatment, VRE infections often occur in hospitals.

VRE is highly resistant to almost all available antibiotics. It is also hardy and has been known to survive for weeks on hospital-room surfaces that cleaning staff might have missed.

ESBL-Producing Bacteria

ESBL stands for extended-spectrum beta-lactamase. Beta-lactamases are enzymes, and ESBLs are enzymes that destroy antibiotics like penicillin. Bacteria that produce ESBLs are, naturally enough, resistant to those antibiotics. ESBLs are most commonly produced by two bacteria: *Escherichia coli* (*E. coli* for short) and *Klebsiella pneumoniae*. But ESBL enzymes can also be found in bacteria such as *Salmonella, Proteus, Morganella, Enterobacter, Citrobacter, Serratia,* and *Pseudomonas.* When the bacteria that cause disease also produce ESBLs, they are pretty hard to get rid of.

In most cases, the body successfully fights off ESBL-producing bacteria. But because of the enzymes' ability to destroy antibiotics, people with weak immune systems are at risk. This includes children, the elderly, and people with serious illnesses.

ESBL-producing bacteria are spread through feces, either by self-infection or direct contact with the feces of an infected person. It can, for example, spread from patient to patient on the hands of health-care workers or the patients themselves. That's why hospitals and homes for seniors are particularly prone to outbreaks.

Pseudomonas aeruginosa

The *Pseudomonas aeruginosa* strain of bacteria is notorious for its resistance to antibiotics and is therefore a particularly dangerous and dreaded pathogen.

It is common in soil and water and on vegetation. It is also found on the skin of some healthy people. Within a hospital setting, *P. aeruginosa* can be found in disinfectants, respiratory equipment, food, sinks, taps, and mops. It is constantly reintroduced into a disinfected environment through fruits, plants, and vegetables, as well as by visitors and by patients transferred from other facilities. It is spread from patient to patient on the hands of hospital personnel, by patients coming in direct contact with contaminated items, and by the ingestion of contaminated food and water.

Pseudomonas aeruginosa is an opportunistic pathogen, meaning that it exploits some break in a patient's natural defenses to initiate an infection. It causes urinary tract infections, respiratory system infections, dermatitis, soft tissue infections, bacteremia, bone and joint infections, gastrointestinal infections, and a variety of systemic infections, particularly in patients with severe burns, as well as in cancer and AIDS patients, who have compromised immune systems. *P. aeruginosa* infection is in fact a very serious problem in patients hospitalized with cancer, cystic fibrosis, and burns. The fatality rate in these patients is 50 percent.

Only a few antibiotics are effective against *P. aeruginosa*, including fluoroquinolones, gentamicin, and imipenem, and even these antibiotics are not effective against all strains of the bacteria. The futility of treating *P. aeruginosa* infections with antibiotics is most graphically illustrated in cystic fibrosis patients: virtually all of them eventually become infected with a strain that is so antibiotic-resistant that it can't be treated.

ASKED AND ANSWERED: In 2007, British health authorities ordered male doctors in direct contact with patients to stop wearing neckties, on the grounds that ties are rarely cleaned and can therefore be prime infection transmitters.

Clostridium difficile

Clostridium difficile—C. difficile for short (and often abbreviated verbally to "c-diff")—upsets the normal balance of healthy bacteria in the digestive system, causing extreme diarrhea and cramps, as well as other complications. It often affects people who have been taking antibiotics, especially broad-spectrum antibiotics which kill a wide variety of bacteria. Not only is this hospital infection fairly common and dangerous, it can be humiliating for patients because it often requires them to be diapered.

The *C. difficile* strain of bacteria has been around for a long time, but it made headlines a few years ago because a study of Quebec hospitals reported a dramatically higher rate of death in people with the infection it causes. Instead of the usual average annual hospital death rate of 1.5 percent among all patients, some hospitals had a death rate of 8.5 percent among those who became infected. Other statistics since have confirmed that this one can be a killer. Rates at which people become infected have also increased recently, and researchers are now worried that an even more deadly strain of *C. difficile* has arrived.

Clostridium difficile doesn't normally cause trouble for healthy people, but for people taking antibiotics it becomes a problem when it takes over in the colon or large intestine, causing diarrhea and damaging the colon. Most of the recent cases of *C. difficile*-caused infections have been reported in hospitals and nursing homes; both are places where patients typically receive the broad-spectrum antibiotics that increase the risk of *C. difficile* infection. The infection is easily spread from person to person through contaminated instruments and dirty hands.

Symptoms of *C. difficile* infection include watery diarrhea, diarrhea containing blood or mucus, abdominal pain and cramps, fever, chills, and rapid heartbeat. For mild cases, the typical treatment is to stop the antibiotics. The balance of healthy bacteria in the colon is usually restored, and that gets rid of the problem. For more severe cases, the original antibiotics are stopped and new antibiotics (usually metronidazole or vancomycin) are started. These two antibiotics target *C. dif-ficile* itself to help the body fight the infection. In very severe cases where antibiotics don't work, surgery may be needed.

S M A R T   M O V E S : **Avoiding *C. difficile* Infection**

- Wash your hands thoroughly with soap and water after using the washroom, and wash them again before and after handling food or medications. If you leave your loved one's room for a coffee break or for any other purpose, wash your hands immediately when you return.

- Encourage visitors, including hospital staff, to follow the same hand-washing routine.

- Watch your loved one for any signs of abdominal discomfort, and notify the nurse immediately if your loved one reports an irregular bowel movement.

- Normally, people suffering with *C. difficile* infection are placed in isolation. Staff and visitors are required to wear disposable protective clothing—an awkward outfit that makes everyone look like an alien—until the infection goes away. Be sensitive to your loved one's physical and emotional discomfort throughout the ordeal, but never touch your loved one without wearing disposable gloves. Even after the defeat of the bad bacteria, infection can recur.

Discharge

Your participation in your loved one's care should extend to discharge planning. After all, isn't going home the goal you, your loved one, and the hospital staff all share?

Sometimes discharge from the hospital seems to happen all at once and in a hurry. But effective discharge planning is a process, not a single event. It should take into account what a patient needs for a smooth transition from one level of care to another. Remember—discharge from a hospital doesn't mean that your loved one is fully recovered. It simply means that a doctor has determined that the patient's condition is stable and that the patient no longer needs hospital-level care.

For a variety of reasons, you may think that your loved one isn't ready to go home. If you disagree with the doctor, you can appeal the decision to the hospital management. If your arguments for keeping your loved one hospitalized are valid and reasonable, most hospital managers will comply. They're not about to invite the bad press that could potentially follow a decision to toss someone out while they still need care.

If your appeal doesn't work or if you want to make a formal complaint about some aspect of your loved one's care while in the hospital, use the Hospital Complaints Process quick-reference sheet as a guide; see it in this chapter and at the back of the book.

Although only a doctor can authorize a hospital discharge, a lot of other people are involved in working out the details of the plan. As the patient's caregiver, you should consider yourself one of the most important. You alone have essential information about your loved one's home situation. And you probably already have a pretty good idea of your own caregiving capabilities because you've been involved in care from the outset.

Be Prepared

Early in your loved one's stay, you should make a point of finding the discharge planner and introducing yourself. That person could be a nurse, a social worker, an administrator, or someone with another title. It's important for you to know who this person is and to understand what they can and cannot do. The discharge planner is responsible for making sure that the plan for your loved one's discharge is "safe and adequate." Although that official term could be open to interpretation, it is generally understood to mean that (1) the patient is going to a place that doesn't present immediate dangers to his or her health and well-being, and (2) realistic plans have been made for appropriate follow-up care.

Discharge planning is a short-term strategy to get your loved one out of the hospital. It's not a blueprint for the future. Your loved one's

Hospital Complaints Process
(Make as many photocopies as you need.)

Complaint Specifics
  Date of Incident:
  Time of Incident:
  Place of Incident:
Communication (lack of information, misunderstanding, or inappropriate communication):
Patient Care (medical error; personal or clinical treatment of patient):
Patient Services (food, hospital room, sanitation, or infection-control lapses):
Hospital Policy (visiting hours, other policies, surgery cancelled because of lack of beds):
Other (health provider conduct, treatment of caregiver, treatment of other family members or visitors, etc.):

Steps to Take
1. If the scope of the complaint is limited to the hospital unit housing the patient, discuss the complaint with:
  Charge Nurse (name):
    Date of Conversation:
  Satisfactory Resolution?   Yes   No   Explain:
If not satisfied, contact:
  Unit/Program Manager (name):
    Date of Conversation:
  Satisfactory Resolution?   Yes   No   Explain:
2. If the complaint could affect others or has not been resolved, register a written complaint with the senior executive responsible for patient relations (name):
3. Outline your concerns clearly, using the 5 W's: who, when, where, what (or how), and why.
4. Copy the hospital CEO and the unit/program manager on all correspondence.

What to Expect

1. A letter or phone call acknowledging your complaint.
2. An investigation involving all parties, including interviews with the patient, family, and staff and perhaps a review of the patient's medical chart.
3. A report that may include the following recommendations:

    Making a patient relations specialist available for ongoing consultation with the family

    Providing feedback to the staff involved and providing training if necessary

    Outlining specific actions for improvement
4. Follow-up by the management to confirm compliance with all the recommendations.

condition may improve or worsen over time. And you may not be able to sustain the intense level of caregiving that's required at the outset. Even though no one can predict what your loved one's needs will be weeks or months after discharge, you should think about the long term as much as possible. You may be able to build services into the immediate plan that will be important further down the road.

Many health-care providers say that discharge planning should begin on the day of admission. That's good in theory, but from-the-start planning is not always practical. If your loved one's admission to the hospital was for a scheduled surgery, for instance, the doctor no doubt gave you some idea of how long the hospital stay would be. In such cases, discharge planning can start even before admission.

But if the hospital stay was unplanned, if it came about because of an accident or a heart attack, you may not know for days or even weeks how long your loved one will be in the hospital or what his or her condition will be. Still, it's a good idea to start thinking about the options as soon as the outcome becomes a little clear. Try to avoid making major decisions under pressure, and don't accept a discharge plan that you're uncomfortable with. The plan has to work for you, too. Most of the time, you can negotiate an acceptable arrangement with your loved one and the discharge planner.

There could be disagreements, of course. Your loved one may want to go home as quickly as possible—maybe too quickly. Or the hospital may need the bed. As the family caregiver, you may have to balance your loved one's preferences and the hospital's needs against the hard realities of the situation. Since your loved one may have unrealistic expectations about what he or she can do without help, you might ask a nurse or doctor to evaluate your loved one and explain to both of you together what your loved one will and won't be able to do. This assessment will help you determine how much care will be needed immediately after discharge and for the first few weeks thereafter.

The strategy for post-hospital care should take into account the following fundamental points:

> your loved one's current condition
> any changes in your loved one's condition that may be a result of

the original reason for hospitalization, like lingering physical or
mental impairment because of a stroke

any likely symptoms, problems, or changes that may occur once
your loved one is at home

your loved one's needs, the caregiver's needs, and any adjustments that must be made to meet these needs

the potential impact of caregiving on the caregiver, warning signs
of stress, and options for reducing stress

SMART MOVES: **Discharge Checklist**

- Ask for specific instructions. These should include any treatment directions as well as diet or lifestyle changes that you and
your loved one may need to incorporate at home.

- Ask for a list of medications upon discharge. If there are any new
medications, request all available information about them, including potential side effects.

- Make sure you understand which of your usual home medications your loved one should continue and which ones to stop.
The hospital pharmacist may be helpful in screening the whole
list to make sure all the medications can be taken together safely.

- Give your family doctor the new list of medications so that your
loved one's record will be updated.

- Ask if there's a plan for follow-up medical appointments and how
to schedule them.

- Keep a copy of the medications list with you or your loved one at
all times so that it's available for office visits or for health-care
providers in case of an emergency.

- Check your medical insurance for at-home coverage.

If your loved one has medical insurance, you will need to know
what's covered. Patients and their families are often shocked to find that
insurance won't pay for many services and items needed at home that
are routinely provided in the hospital. Unless your loved one has specific long-term care insurance (and very few people do), many home-

Agenda for a Meeting to Plan Patient Discharge
(Make as many photocopies as you need.)

Name of Discharge Planner:

Date and Time of Meeting:

Place of Meeting:

Date of Anticipated Discharge:

Condition of Patient (caregiver's opinion):   Poor   Fair   Good
    In the caregiver's opinion, is the patient ready for discharge?

    If no, state reasons:

**What an Effective and Comprehensive Discharge Plan
Should Include**
1. The continuing care services the patient will need, including medical
treatments, medical transportation, and homemaker services.

2. Detailed information about the services that have been arranged.

3. Names, addresses, and phone numbers of the service providers.

4. A schedule outlining when at-home nursing or rehabilitation services will begin.

5. Medications that the patient will need and clear instructions for their use.

6. Information about special diets and treatments, including dietary restrictions, if any.

7. The detailed schedule for any of the patient's follow-up medical appointments.

8. Advice on what to monitor at home, including fever or any bleeding, and who to call in the event of an emergency.

9. A detailed explanation of the process of appealing a discharge decision, including staff members to contact and forms to complete.

Notes

care supplies and home-care aides or attendants will not be covered beyond an initial short-term period—if at all.

Even though your primary concern is your loved one's health, it makes sense to find out early on what follow-up care will be paid for and what the family will be responsible for. The discharge planner or a social worker can help you get started, but you may also want to talk to others who have been in the same situation. Some short-term home care—for, say, a few weeks or a month—may be covered, but even that's not guaranteed. Coverage may also depend on your loved one's progress at home and other factors. Although the hospital discharge planner may not be able to give you all the information you need about home-care benefits, you can at least be directed to home-care agencies and other community resources.

The Agenda for a Meeting to Plan Patient Discharge quick-reference sheet provides a useful list of information to collect and questions to ask; you can find it in this chapter and at the back of the book. Look through it, use it to guide you through the discharge process, and fill it in and keep it as a record of the plan for post-hospital care. You can use the Medical/Surgical Follow-up Appointments quick-reference sheet to enter appointments made for follow-up care; it's also nearby and at the back of the book.

Be Persistent

Given the costs of at-home care and the usual lack of insurance coverage, the financial picture may be discouraging, but don't give up trying to nail down a post-hospital care plan. There are lots of ways to make the case with insurers that the care your loved one needs is "medically necessary" or that your loved one's condition continues to improve (a requirement to carry on with physical or occupational therapy). You may be able to justify the need for durable medical equipment, such as a special hospital bed and mattress at home.

You might be surprised at the adjustments that need to be made to assure a safe house for the returning patient—everything from a bell for your loved one to ring for help to a wheelchair ramp. Take a look

Medical/Surgical Follow-up Appointments
(Make as many photocopies as you need.)

Name of Physician or Surgeon:

Address:

Phone Number:

Pager:

Date and Time of Appointment:

Special Instructions:

Notes:

Name of Physician or Surgeon:

Address:

Phone Number:

Pager:

Date and Time of Appointment:

Special Instructions:

Notes:

around your house, and use the Home Preparation Checklist quick-reference sheet provided to help you think through the adjustments you might need to make—and the requests you might make of your insurance carrier. You can review the checklist in this chapter or at the back of the book.

A word of caution: If someone tells you that Medicare (or any provincial or state insurance plan) "won't pay for it," don't stop there. Check it out yourself by calling the appropriate agency or insurance provider—and keep careful records of all conversations, including the names of the people you speak with and when. Insurance coverage decisions are often flexible; indeed, you may need to document different interpretations that different people have given you. Maybe another member of the family could take on this single task. Chasing down bureaucrats can take enormous time and energy.

Be Realistic

You want to do what's best for your loved one, but you also have to consider all your other obligations. You may be able to take some time off from work, but not enough, and perhaps it's not feasible to quit your job. You may be able to provide some care, but not all of it. You may have health problems of your own that prevent you from handling some kinds of care. Your other family responsibilities may limit your availability.

Hospital staff might assume that because you've been a faithful companion to your loved one in the hospital, you will now be available full-time for future care. If that's not the case, you need to say so—firmly and consistently. A discharge plan that's based on faulty assumptions or incomplete information is not going to work. With the help of one of the health-care providers who has looked after your loved one, compile a list of all the tasks that will have to be done when your loved one leaves the hospital. Then be honest with yourself and check off only those that you're certain you can undertake. Make another list that contains the names of people and resources who can help provide care. In any case, don't assume you can manage everything all by yourself.

Home Preparation Checklist
(Make as many photocopies as you need.)

Safety Check

    A ramp to the front door to accommodate a wheelchair or a walker?

    A clear path through each room, with no rugs or raised room dividers to trip over and no slippery floors?

    Furniture rearranged to ease navigation?

    Handrails to help move from one room to another?

    A raised toilet seat for easier sitting?

    Grab bars near the toilet and bathtub for safety in standing and sitting?

    Non-skid mats on the bathroom floor and in the bathtub to prevent slipping and falling?

    Nightlights for safety in moving around at night?

    Working smoke alarms and fire extinguishers throughout the home?

    Emergency numbers—fire, hospital, 911—and contact numbers in a convenient location?

Special Equipment Check

    A hospital bed or other special type of bed?

    Walker? Cane? Wheelchair?

    Bedside commode?

    Lift?

    Oxygen?

Mobility Check

    Is a ramp needed on exterior stairs?

    Will a wheelchair fit through doorways?

    Is it easy to walk or move from room to room without running into furniture?

Communication Check

    Get a cordless speaker phone with speed dial, making it possible to call for emergency help with one push of a button and avoid compromising the safety of your loved one?

Get a phone with a large digital display for easy reading, plus a ring and voice enhancer, if your loved one has a vision or hearing problem?

Get a fully charged cell phone if you and your loved one will be spending time outside the home?

Install a medical or home alert system making it possible to summon help with the push of a button if you will occasionally leave your loved one alone?

Get an intercom or baby monitor in order to listen to your loved one when you are in another room?

Get a hand bell or buzzer that your loved one can use to ring for help?

Notes

By watching carefully while your loved one was in the hospital, you've learned most of the techniques that are important for at-home care. That's why it is important to be involved in your loved one's care all the way through the hospital stay. You may even have had a chance to practice some of the clinical routines and techniques under supervision. Hospital staff won't have any extra time to train you. They may toss a list of care tasks at you as you and your loved on are on the way out the door, so be sure to make comprehensive notes as you go along. Include instructions on using special equipment and tips on dispensing medications.

Making full use of the quick-reference sheets will help you cover the details. Even if you're not going to provide all the care at home yourself, it's important that you understand how the care should be done so that you can instruct or supervise others.

Don't be afraid to say that you cannot or do not want to perform certain tasks, such as tending to personal hygiene or cleansing wounds. Remember that you're a family member, not a professional. You shouldn't have to do anything that interferes with your unique relationship with your loved one. Why should this journey be any rougher for both of you than it has to be?

9
Hospice
Dying with Dignity

Although miracle drugs and space-age surgery persuade us to expect cures for all that ails us, you may one day hear these unwelcome words: "I'm sorry, but there's nothing more we can do. You might want to start thinking about palliative or hospice care."

In a gentle way, you've just been told that your loved one will not recover. The cancer is incurable. The heart or kidney or liver failure is irreversible. The lungs are not recovering, and the breathing is labored. All the normal treatment options have been tried and are no longer working. So your loved one could be facing death—maybe not today or next week or even next month, but time is running out.

Confusion is added to your shock and grief. What's palliative care? What's hospice care? What's the difference between them?

The confusion is understandable. The terms are often used interchangeably, probably because both are associated with end-of-life care and because both have the same goal—to relieve the suffering of seriously ill patients for whom conventional treatment methods—such as chemotherapy and dialysis—have failed. Palliative-care patients may not be in imminent danger of dying, however. In fact, palliative care is sometimes offered in combination with aggressive or investigational treatments that could even carry the possibility of a cure. A lot of hospitals offer palliative care, and these typically have a limited number of beds specifically assigned for that purpose.

Hospice care, on the other hand, is normally delivered outside the hospital and in the community. It's an option for patients who have a terminal diagnosis and who have stopped active treatment because there's no benefit to continuing. They are expected to die. They can die at home or in a hospice building that's large enough to accommodate resident patients. Although palliative-care measures may be used with some hospice patients, they are usually deployed to ease discomfort and improve quality of life. For hospice patients there is no prospect of a cure.

In many cases, patients begin with in-hospital palliative care and then transfer to a hospice.

Palliative care is a fairly new medical specialty, but hospice care goes back to the Middle Ages, when monks offered shelter and food to pilgrims debilitated by grueling journeys. Irish nuns adapted that spirit of hospitality in the late nineteenth century. By opening a facility in Dublin to care for the dying and their families, they were bucking a medical trend. In a society enthralled with scientific and industrial progress, doctors dismissed people with incurable diseases as broken machines, unresponsive to treatment and therefore uninteresting. The charitable nuns were on their own.

In the 1960s hospice care got a major boost from a British nurse who also happened to be a doctor. Cicely Saunders revisited the ancient concept, refined its core principles into a sophisticated care strategy grounded in solid medical principles, and gave it an important role that went far beyond kind words and clean sheets. She argued that dying is really about living as fully as possible—and that science and the human heart could partner to help it happen.

Saunders, who is credited with launching the modern hospice movement, founded the world's first freestanding hospice in London in 1967. She did it because she knew that some terminal patients wouldn't want to die in a hospital but didn't have the personal support or resources to end their lives peacefully at home. Consistent with her beliefs, Saunders committed St. Christopher's Hospice to providing care that responded to a patient's "total pain"—her term for the physical, spiritual, psychological, and social pain of the dying patient. She emphasized a multidisciplinary approach to caring for the dying, the regular use of opioids like morphine to control physical pain, and respectful regard for the deep suffering also endured by the patient's family. Her work infuses hospice care today, even though some hospital nurses and doctors still believe that morphine shouldn't be administered to the dying because it's addictive. That irony was not lost on Saunders, who argued that effective pain management is a major key to assuring comfort in a patient's final days.

Hospice caregivers pay close attention to the whole person—to the whole range of human needs invoked in the course of dying. In that sense, hospice care is both broader and deeper than palliative care: it's based on a set of beliefs that aren't just clinical. Like the pilgrims of the Middle Ages, hospice patients are encouraged to reflect on their lives, to seek meaning in them, to accept that death is the next phase of existence.

ASKED AND ANSWERED: The first U.S. hospice opened in Branford, Connecticut, in 1974. The first Canadian hospice opened in Quebec City in 1985. There are now more than four thousand hospices in North America, with 90 percent of patients receiving hospice care at home.

Hospice Care
Who Cares?

Hospice care was developed in response to the needs of the dying patient, but the patient's family is also integrated into the care strategy. Including family members is not a matter of mushy sentiment. Family members are often the principal caregivers for hospice patients, especially those housed at home, and they may need support from hospice staff and volunteers to fill the role effectively. Compassion is another hallmark of hospice care—compassion not only for the patient but also for those who are threatened with the loss of a loved one. Many hos-

pices make bereavement support available to families for up to a year after the death of a patient.

The professional part of the team usually has the following core
members: a hospice doctor (usually on call), a registered nurse, a nursing assistant, a social worker, and a chaplain. The patient's own doctor
could be part of the team along with the hospice doctor, and homemak-
ers, home health aides, physical and occupational therapists, speech
therapists, dietitians, and others may join in along the way. Volunteers
are essential to the team. They undertake such load-lightening tasks as
shuttling patients to and from doctors' appointments and, at many hospices, help give family caregivers breaks by transporting patients out of
the home for the day and into a group space where they can socialize
with other patients. That break is called respite care, and it helps patients and family caregivers alike.

Although there are now freestanding hospices like the original St.
Christopher's all over the world, hospice has come to be associated
largely with the provision of care in the patient's own home, with death
normally occurring there instead of a hospital—and often in a hospital-
type bed provided specifically for end-of-life care. But hospice isn't defined by place. In addition to home, hospice patients can be temporarily cared for in hospitals, outpatient clinics, and nursing homes and
other extended-care facilities. In fact, patients sometimes move among
these settings as their conditions or their family needs change, even
choosing to spend some time in a hospital or nursing home to give family caregivers some needed time off.

Who Pays?

In Canada, most provinces cover all or some portion of hospice care,
but there are variables and conditions, so it's advisable to check with
the Ministry of Health in your own jurisdiction for details.

In the United States, although most private insurance plans offer
coverage for hospice care, Medicare pays for most hospice services, accounting for about 70 percent of the total cost. Medicare also certifies
most hospices in the United States. About 80 percent of those who use

hospice care are over the age of sixty-five, but Medicare hospice benefits are available to anyone eligible for Medicare Part A, although there are some exclusions. The most fundamental exclusion disqualifies patients who seek curative or aggressive treatment for a terminal condition, but they are eligible to return to the Medicare coverage they had if they abandon that kind of treatment before entering hospice. Medicare paid out $90 billion in claims in 2006. Given rapid medical advances, there is growing pressure to allow hospice patients to opt for treatments that might restore some to health, which would offer a margin of hope to those patients and perhaps ease the financial burden on Medicare. Even now, Medicare will continue to cover treatments for health problems unrelated to the patient's terminal illness as long as a patient is in hospice. Medicaid also covers hospice care in most states for those who are eligible for that program. Be sure to check with Medicare before making decisions, though. Regulations change.

Choosing a Hospice—or Not

As an end-of-life care choice, hospice still isn't universally embraced. The decision to enter a hospice feels too final for many patients and family members, no matter how grim the prognosis may be. Some see going into hospice as giving up—giving up on the patient, giving up on efforts to prolong life, giving up hope. Nor is every experience with hospice care a happy one. Because all facilities struggle to balance patients' needs with financial imperatives, mistakes and omissions are bound to happen. Money for health care is short everywhere, and hospices aren't exempt from the pressure of just trying to keep their doors open.

Many people share the misconception that hospices advocate euthanasia—that they actively work to hasten death. That view probably arises from the hospice requirement that patients decline treatment that's intended to cure, as well as from the scheduled use of analgesics while patients are in hospice. No one has to wait until they are in severe pain to get relief from it. Advocates of hospice care argue that the hospice seeks neither to hasten nor to prolong dying but to assist patients in living as comfortably as possible until death arrives naturally. The assumption that links hospice with euthanasia frustrates many who work in hospice, not only because it makes some patients and families reluctant to choose hospice but also because it runs counter to everything that hospice is about. Cicely Saunders herself strongly opposed euthanasia and saw hospice as a positive alternative to it—as a way to manage dying (including pain) so effectively that there would be no need to consider euthanasia. She concluded from her experience that dying patients feared pain above all, and campaigned to free them from needless suffering.

If you and your loved one discuss hospice and decide in favor of it, your doctor or the hospital should be able to provide a list of local hospices. There's also a short list of Web sites and hospices in the Resources section at the back of the book. Before you make a choice of hospice, you should seek answers to some basic questions:

Does the hospice serve your own area?

(In the United States:) Is the hospice licensed and Medicare/Medicaid certified?

Does the hospice provide the services you want and need?

What does the hospice expect from you and the caregiver support system?

Will your insurance plan or health plan work with the hospice?

Does the hospice have a support program for caregivers?

Are inpatient and respite care provided? Where?

Is the hospice's position on resuscitation, hydration, and antibiotics consistent with yours?

What out-of-pocket expenses should you anticipate?

Is there a sliding-scale payment plan for services not covered by insurance?

Once you've narrowed your search for a hospice to a couple of possibilities, use the Questions When Choosing a Hospice quick-reference sheet to guide you to a final decision; you can find it nearby and at the back of the book.

Questions When Choosing a Hospice
(Make as many photocopies as you need.)

Patient's Needs and Wishes
How do the hospice staff, working with the patient and loved ones,
honor the patient's wishes?

Family Involvement and Support
Are family caregivers given the information and training they need to
care for the patient at home?

What services does the hospice offer to help the patient and loved ones
deal with grief and loss?

Is respite care (relief for the caregiver) available?

Are loved ones told what to expect in the dying process and what happens after the patient's death?

What bereavement services are available after the patient dies?

Physician and Staff
What is the role of the patient's physician once hospice care begins?

How will the hospice physician oversee the patient's care and work
with the patient's doctor?

How many patients does each hospice staff member care for?

Volunteers
What services do volunteers offer?

What screening and type of training do hospice volunteers receive?

Comfort and Pain Management
Do the hospice staff regularly discuss and routinely evaluate pain control and symptom management with patients and families?

Do the hospice staff respond immediately to requests for additional
pain medication?

What specialty or expanded programs does the hospice offer?

How does the hospice meet the spiritual and emotional needs of the patient and the family?

After-Hours Care

How quickly do hospice staff respond to after-hours emergencies?

Are a chaplain and a social worker available after hours? Are others?

How are calls and visits handled when death occurs?

Various Care Settings

How does the hospice provide services for residents in nursing homes and other such care settings?

How does the hospice work with hospitals and other facilities during the course of the patient's stay?

What will happen if care cannot be managed at home?

Quality of Care

What credentials do the hospice staff have? Do they have special credentials in their specialties?

Is the hospice program certified and licensed?

What other kind of accreditation or certification does the hospice program have? How about its staff?

What measures does the hospice take to ensure quality?

Paying for Hospice Care

Are all of the costs of hospice care covered by the patient's health insurance?

What services will the patient have to pay for out of pocket? Are any services provided at no charge?

Responses to Dying

Veteran hospice workers will confirm that everyone copes with dying in different ways. That's no surprise. We live differently, so why shouldn't we die differently? Still, the dying have common ground, apart from the obvious. For them all, to die peacefully and to die knowing that their life has had meaning are important. In that sense, hospice seeks to help provide a good death. You might wonder what death can possibly be good. As hospice defines it, a good death is one that has positive benefits for the dying person and for family and friends. More to the point, a good death is a central goal of hospice care.

ASKED AND ANSWERED: When Cicely Saunders opened her landmark London hospice in 1967, almost all of her patients were dying of cancer. In 2006, only 44 percent of U.S. hospice patients had cancer, according to the National Hospice and Palliative Care Organization. Heart disease ranked second to cancer, at 12 percent.

No one should try to tell people who are dying what's best for them. That's why it is important to find out where our loved ones want to die, how they want their pain managed, what they want health-care providers to do, and how much they want the family to be involved in their care. Do they want specific funeral arrangements to be made? Do they want celebrations for holidays and birthdays to continue while they are in hospice? Gently urge your loved one to communicate such wishes. If you can begin to think of hospice as a shift in life rather than a move toward death, your loved one has a better chance of easing into the transition. But remember that your loved one needs to feel in charge, as physically diminished as his or her life may be. People rightly cherish their independence, even when they are dying. Your loved one shouldn't feel disenfranchised by the process.

Dying affects many dimensions of life: physical, psychological, social, and spiritual. Hospice care deals with all of them. You will want to watch for the ways dying affects your loved one along all these dimensions. Even the most attentive nurse may not catch significant responses.

Physical Responses

Alleviating physical symptoms is the first challenge in end-of-life care. Pain, difficulty breathing, gastrointestinal disturbances, delirium, agitation, fatigue, and anorexia (prolonged loss of appetite) require care that aims to control or relieve these symptoms so that the patient has as much physical function as possible.

Caregiver opportunity: Be alert to physical discomfort in your loved one, even if it's not openly acknowledged. Someone who is dying may assume that discomfort is a constant part of the process even though relief is not only possible but desirable.

Psychological Responses

When facing the end of life, most people experience a variety of psychological symptoms. Sadness, depression, anxiety, and other such feelings are normal. They reflect all the losses felt by the dying person—loss of energy, loss of the ability to enjoy hobbies and former interests, loss of a future with family and friends. The standard criteria for diagnosing depression cannot usually be applied to the dying person. In those who are terminally ill, feelings of helplessness, hopelessness, worthlessness, and guilt, together with thoughts of suicide, are better indicators. Anxiety is typically tied to worry, apprehension, and fear—for example, worries about being separated from loved ones, concerns about being a burden to others, and fears about a painful death.

Caregiver opportunity: You know the hospice patient—report any unusual reactions or behavior to the nurse.

Social Responses

Once the term *dying* is applied to a person, that person's role or place in all of life's activities often changes. Your loved one may no longer be able to work, to drive, to engage in familiar sports or hobbies. Your loved one may be dependent on you for tasks once routinely undertaken, even down to matters of personal hygiene. Your loved one's role within the family may also change as the family tries to take on tasks once automatically assumed by the dying person. This can lead to feelings of distress, loss, frustration, and depression.

If the dying person is elderly, family members may assume that he or she is ready to die and doesn't need much interaction with others. In some cases, social isolation can result as friends and even family members drift away. Sometimes, too, people don't know what to say to a dying person and, fearing an awkward conversation, duck the chance to visit. But the yearning for intimate social contact doesn't go away just because a person is dying. If anything, it increases—even though the dying person may sometimes appear to be withdrawn or disconnected.

Caregiver opportunity: Talk with your loved one, and facilitate visits from family and friends. Include the loved one in social activities and events as much as possible.

Spiritual Responses

Spiritual care has always been one of the pillars of the hospice movement, even from its earliest days, when providers tacitly understood that spiritual pain can be as intense as physical pain. When people are facing imminent death, they may feel angry and desolate. They often struggle to find a meaning and purpose in life. They need to give love and to receive it. They need to hope. Some people may have solid religious or philosophical beliefs that help them accept death and the experience of dying. Others don't know where to begin.

Religion and spirituality don't necessarily mean the same thing. While spirituality is usually a component of religion, a person doesn't need to be religious to be a spiritual being. Religions usually include certain beliefs and rituals that can comfort adherents when they are dying, but spirituality is much broader. It encompasses existence itself, touching on people's connection with themselves and others, as well as with the universe. Spiritual and religious beliefs can give meaning and purpose to life, not only for the dying person but for everyone personally involved. Both patient and family may be in spiritual turmoil over the impending loss and death. That is common and understandable.

Caregiver opportunity: Give your loved one and yourself time to look back on your life together. Enjoy the memories. Recall what's been significant, and realize that life can continue to be meaningful even in its last stages. Most hospices have chaplains on call, and the best of them are skilled and compassionate listeners who do not proselytize or offer platitudes. If you think a chaplain could be beneficial to your loved one's comfort, find out first if your loved one would welcome a visit, and then make the call.

SMART MOVES: Things to Do and Watch For

- Try to relate to the person, not the illness. That can inspire friends and the rest of your family to behave the same way.

- Be attentive. Undivided attention is the greatest gift you can offer to your dying loved one.

- Keep conversation as normal as possible, remembering that your loved one's mental faculties will probably remain acute unless dementia is involved.

- Listen without judgment. Watch for nonverbal cues, and respect the personal truths your loved one may be discovering. Allow your loved one to express thoughts and fears about dying, and be honest in your responses.

- Don't just think compassionately—act compassionately. Place a cool cloth on a perspiring brow or hold your loved one's hand when fear threatens.

- Create a calm environment. Leave space for silence between you and your loved one. Stillness that demands absolutely nothing except a human presence can be therapeutic.

- Be ready to laugh at shared jokes or experiences. Laughter doesn't have to be abandoned in the face of death. Often it is the healthy thing to do.

- Don't be afraid to let your own fear and anxiety show. If you feel helpless, admit that openly to your loved one. Your honesty can bring you closer together and open freer communication. Sometimes the dying know better than we how they can be helped.

- Remember that you're considered a full partner on the hospice care team, with the same rights and responsibilities as everyone else. That means remaining vigilant. Watch for any pain or discomfort. Be alert to any changes, physical or psychological, in your loved one that could influence care. Tell the nurse immediately if you see anything that puzzles or disturbs you.

Activities

If your loved one spends a lot of time sleeping, don't be concerned. Sleeping is a normal reaction to the analgesics and sedatives that ease pain and discomfort. Sleep is also needed because this business of dying can be exhausting, and there's a good chance your loved one is trying to come to terms internally with it. Should you leave while your loved one is asleep? You don't have to. You can remain, sitting quietly and stroking a hand every now and then to let your loved one know you're there. Once in a while, your loved one may wake up with a sense of urgency and immediately want to share a dream. That, too, is normal. Dreams are part of the struggle to work things out. That moment of sharing is a gift. Treasure it. You may learn something new about this person who's been a familiar part of your life for years.

There will be good days and bad days. There will be moments when your loved one seems to be completely normal, when reality is swept aside, and the vibrant person you remember seems to have returned. When that happens, especially after a long period of apparent decline, it's understandably tempting to believe that some kind of miracle has occurred. Try to remain calm. Don't set yourself up for disappointment. After dozing off, your loved one is likely to wake up as a dying person again.

Visits from family and friends are important, but hospice patients can tire easily from the simple effort of engaging with people. They don't want to disappoint anyone who makes time to visit, so they try to rise to the occasion, which can exhaust their energy. You may have to eventually limit visiting times to only a few minutes. Take your cues from your loved one, even if they aren't spoken out loud.

Things to Do

Much of hospice care comes down to watching and waiting, so you may occasionally wonder whether there's anything else you can do. Although the following activities aren't for everyone, many hospice patients and their families report that they can be beneficial and fun.

JOURNAL WRITING: Keeping a journal of your loved one's closing days can be an effective way to deal with your own grief, but it can also expand to include favorite family stories and recollections, with contributions from everyone. You can encourage your loved one to enter thoughts and comments, even to share feelings about what she or he is going through. The journal can become a memorial to your loved one and to the whole final experience.

FAMILY PHOTOGRAPHS: Family members can select photographs to place in a special album, writing captions next to each one. Young family members may appreciate learning about their family's history. For your loved one, it can help heal and connect.

A COLLECTION OF FAVORITE THINGS: Encourage the family to help organize a collection of the things everyone associates with your loved one, and group them near your loved one's bed so they're easy to see. A baseball or a special recipe or a book can bring a reminiscent smile to everyone's face.

A MEMORY GARDEN: Planting a tree, a bush, or perennial flowers, either in your own backyard or in a public place, can carry your loved one forward in everyone's memory. When a much-loved father named Bill died, the family planted a maple tree that's now a healthy twenty-five feet high. It's affectionately called Bill whenever anyone admires it.

MUSIC: Don't underestimate the power of music to bring ease to a dying person. Music can often be particularly useful near the end of life when communication starts to break down. A word of caution: You may assume that your loved one wants to hear the same music preferred earlier—that, say, a big fan of the Rolling Stones will want to listen to their albums. Near the end of life most people want to hear soothing music, however. Typical choices include classical compositions by Mozart and Bach or gentle environmental sounds like ocean waves and wind and rain. The goal is to relax the dying person and encourage a sense of peace—but if a rock opera is requested, crank it up.

ART: Sometimes people who are dying yearn to put their internal struggle into visual form as a way of helping others and themselves understand what they're going through. Art therapy is based on the principle that individuals project their internal world into visual forms, and you can encourage your loved one to create a painting, a collage, or a simple sketch. Some of what you see may be startling or even disturbing, but it can be a liberating way for your loved one to communicate when words become elusive.

OUTINGS: If your loved one is up to it, plan some short outings— to a local restaurant, a movie, or a local park. Short trips take the focus from the illness to the trip itself and give both of you a fresh perspective.

PETS: Animals have been known to have a therapeutic effect on dying people. If your loved one has always been fond of pets but the family doesn't have one, recruit a neighbor's familiar dog for a brief visit. Even the goofiest dogs tend to behave differently with very ill people, slipping into respectful and sensitive roles that are astonishing to witness. Animal experts claim that pets know instinctively when someone is gravely ill, and they seem to respond with gentle, loving behavior.

Sensations

Your loved one's five senses—touch, smell, taste, sight, and hearing—may appear to be in retreat, but you might try summoning them as a way to connect and comfort. Here are examples of things you can do.

TOUCH: Touching is a powerful way to break the isolation, the loneliness, and the fear of dying. Ask the nurse to assess your loved one, bearing in mind he or she could be in pain and resist being touched. Then ask the nurse to guide you and your family in the use of appropriate touch. In most cases, touching, the most basic human form of contact, can bring a sense of peace.

SMELL: Smells can elicit powerful emotions. Illness will probably change the types of scents that the sick person can tolerate, but your loved one may be able to enjoy mild-smelling lotions and colognes. Natural scents like rosemary and vanilla, a fragrant plant, and a mildly scented candle are usually what are best appreciated. Use caution when incorporating fragrances into end-of-life care, though, because some scents may cause nausea or unpleasant feelings, even if they were once favorites.

TASTE: We all have different taste preferences, and they are usually consistent until we die. Provide food that your loved one has always liked. Tasting and eating together can have symbolic meanings for the patient and the family. But if your loved one no longer wants to eat, don't be upset. That's a choice and probably won't cause undue suffering.

SIGHT: Arrange objects and photographs within easy view. Let the choices represent either meaningful events or people who evoke happy memories. A room with subdued lighting can provide a sense of serenity, and light colors are usually more soothing to the dying person than bright or dark colors.

HEARING: The sense of hearing is often sharp to the very end of life, so special words said at death can still be heard. But it can also be comforting to sit in silence and hold the hand of the dying person.

Signals of Approaching Death

How will you know that the end is close? You can watch for certain signs and symptoms that provide clues that the dying process has entered its final phase. They won't occur identically with every dying person, but the following list will provide some guidance.

Coolness

Your loved one's hands and arms, the feet, and then the legs may become cooler to the touch. At the same time, the skin may acquire a pallor that wasn't there before. This is a normal indication that the circulation of blood to the body's extremities is decreasing and being reserved for the most vital organs. Keep your loved one warm with a regular (not electric) blanket.

Sleeping

Your loved one may spend an increasing amount of time sleeping, appear to be uncommunicative or unresponsive, and be at times difficult to awaken. This is natural and is due in part to changes in the metabolism of the body. Sit with your loved one and hold hands, but don't shake your loved one's hand. Speak softly and naturally. Plan to spend time with your loved one during those times when she or he seems most awake and alert. Don't talk about your loved one in your loved one's presence. Instead, speak to him or her directly as you normally would, even though there may be no response. Never assume that your loved one can't hear—remember that hearing is the last of the senses to be lost.

Disorientation

Your loved one may seem to be confused about the time, the place, and the identity of surrounding people, including those who are close and familiar—including you. Confusion is also due in part to metabolism changes. Identify yourself by name before you speak, rather than compelling your loved one to guess who you are. Speak softly, clearly, and truthfully when you need to communicate something important for the patient's comfort. If you're administering medication, tell your loved one what it's for each time.

Incontinence

Your loved one may lose bladder and bowel control as muscles in those areas begin to relax. Ask your hospice nurse what can be done to protect the bed and keep your loved one clean and comfortable.

Congestion

You may hear gurgling sounds coming from your loved one's chest, and these sounds may become quite loud as time passes. This normal change is caused by the decrease in fluid intake and an inability to cough up normal secretions. Suctioning usually only increases the secretions and causes sharp discomfort. Gently turn your loved one's head to the side and allow gravity to drain the secretions. You may also gently wipe the mouth with a moist cloth. But don't be alarmed—the sound of the congestion doesn't indicate the onset of severe or new pain.

Restlessness

Your loved one may make restless, repetitive motions such as pulling at bed linen or clothing. This often happens and is due in part to the decrease in oxygen circulating to the brain and to metabolism changes. Don't try to impede or restrain these movements. You can have a calming effect by speaking quietly, lightly massaging the forehead, reading to your loved one, or playing soothing music. Some veterans of hospice care claim that restlessness is also a sign of unfinished business, and perhaps they're right. If you feel that way, ask hospice staff to help your loved one gain a measure of peace and acceptance.

Urine Decrease

Your loved one's urine output normally decreases near the end, and it may become tea colored. That concentrated urine is due to decreased fluid intake and decreased circulation through the kidneys. Ask the nurse to determine whether a catheter is needed.

Lost Appetite

Your loved one may lose appetite and want little or no food or fluid. In the final stages before death, the body begins to conserve the energy normally used for eating and drinking and digesting. Don't try to force food or drink into your loved one or use guilt to manipulate your loved one into choking something down. This will only make your loved one uncomfortable. Small chips of ice, frozen Gatorade, or frozen juice may be refreshing in the mouth. If your loved one is still able to swallow, you may be able to give fluids in small amounts by oral syringe. Ask the nurse for guidance. Glycerin swabs may help keep the mouth and lips moist and comfortable. A cool, damp washcloth on the forehead may also increase physical comfort.

Change in Breathing Pattern

Your loved one's regular breathing pattern may change to a different one that consists of shallow breaths followed by no breathing for a period of time that can vary in length from a few seconds to a minute. This is called Cheyne-Stokes breathing, a pattern named after the two doctors who identified it in the nineteenth century. It usually alarms the family but apparently causes no discomfort to the patient. Your loved one may also experience periods of rapid and shallow breathing that sounds like panting. Both patterns are very common and indicate decreased circulation in the internal organs. Elevating the head or turning your loved one onto his or her side may bring comfort. Hold your loved one's hand. Speak gently.

Visionlike Experiences

Your loved one may claim to have spoken to people who have already died or may look at things in the room that are not visible to you. This doesn't necessarily mean that your loved one is hallucinating or having a drug reaction. Your loved one is beginning to detach from this life. Don't contradict, explain away, belittle, or argue about what your loved one claims to see or hear. Accept that the experience is real to your loved one—but if it frightens him or her, explain that it's normal.

Withdrawal

Your loved one may seem unresponsive, withdrawn. or in a coma-like state. This indicates preparation for release, for detachment from surroundings and relationships, the start of letting go. Since hearing remains intact all the way to the end, speak to your loved one in your normal tone of voice, always identifying yourself by name when you speak. Hold his or her hand, and say whatever you need to say that will help your loved one let go.

Decreased Socialization

As death approaches, your loved one's world will probably shrink by choice to include very few people—perhaps only one. This is another sign of readiness to go. All your loved one will want at that point is affirmation and support.

Letting Go

Dying people may not verbalize it, but they often seek permission to go. They normally try to hold on, even though staying prolongs their discomfort, because they want to be sure that those left behind will be all right. You may have to place your own grief and yearning to one side and speak the words your loved one needs to hear before letting go. Saying them may be the hardest thing you ever have to do, but know that they will probably give more comfort than all of the drugs and painkillers put together.

When your loved one is ready to die and you're able to let go, you can say good-bye. That's important. Actually saying good-bye is your final gift. Remember, the words will be heard and will ease the final release. Don't be afraid to cry. You don't have to hide your tears from your loved one. You don't have to apologize or pretend. Now, in this moment, you are both letting go of each other.

How will you know when your loved one has died? The signs of death include such things as no breathing, no heartbeat, release of the bladder and the bowels, no response, eyelids slightly open, pupils enlarged, eyes fixed on a certain spot, no blinking, jaw relaxed, mouth slightly open. A hospice nurse will be available to help you confirm your loved one's condition before notifying the hospice doctor. The police don't have to be called.

There's no hurry. The body doesn't have to be moved until you're ready. You can sit quietly by your loved one if you like, and invite other family members to join you. If family members want to assist in preparing the body by bathing or dressing it, you can encourage that, too.

You may be exhausted and inconsolable right now, but try to hold to a truth that spans the arc of bodily failure and death. You have helped give your loved one a good death, and that realization will grow as your pain gradually eases and your own life moves forward.

Cicely Saunders was eighty-seven when she died in 2005, in the London hospice that she founded. In an earlier interview with the BBC, she explained why she had made hospice her life's work. "I once asked a man who knew he was dying what he needed above all in those who were caring for him. He said, 'For someone to look as if they are trying to understand me.'" Saunders said, "Indeed, it is impossible to understand fully another person, but I never forgot that he did not ask for success. He only asked that someone should care enough to try."

Whether in hospital or hospice, that's a very good starting point for the people we entrust with our lives.

A Hospital Lexicon

What Does That Mean? Terms for Medical Conditions, Common Hospital Procedures, and Other Health-Related Matters

Hospital-speak may sound like a foreign language to anyone outside the health-care industry, but you will need to understand what the medical professionals are saying if you spend time at a hospital patient's bedside. Like most professionals, health-care providers use oral and written shorthand to communicate clinical information to one another, making it even harder for outsiders to understand what is going on. When written, certain abbreviations can look like hieroglyphics to the uninitiated. When spoken, they can baffle and confuse. You may hear them at the patient's bedside or see them scrawled on prescriptions, doctors' orders, admission forms, medical charts, clinical assessments, or diagnostic reports. The list of terms and abbreviations given here is not comprehensive, and many definitions have been simplified, but it should help you figure out what the care providers are telling your loved one, you, and each other.

ABDOMINAL HYSTERECTOMY *See* hysterectomy.

ABDOMINOSCOPY Assessment using a laparoscope, which is inserted into one or more small incisions to examine the abdominal cavity. *See also* laparoscopy.

ABNORMAL A term used to describe a variance from the norm in anything from behavior to a test result.

ABSCESS A local accumulation of pus anywhere in the body.

AC Before meals.

ACTIVITIES OF DAILY LIVING (ADL) The things we normally do every day, including activities for self-care, such as feeding, bathing, dressing, and grooming ourselves. The ability or inability to perform ADLs can be used as a very practical measure of ability/disability in many disorders.

ACUTE ILLNESS Any illness characterized by the rapid onset of signs and symptoms that are usually severe and that impair the normal functioning of the patient.

ACUTE OTITIS MEDIA Inflammation of the middle ear that typically causes fluid to accumulate in the middle ear, giving signs or symptoms of ear infection: a bulging eardrum, usually with pain, or a perforated eardrum, often with drainage of purulent material (pus).

ACUTE RESPIRATORY DISTRESS SYNDROME (ARDS) The sudden and devastating onset of respiratory failure—the lungs stop functioning normally and mechanical ventilation is needed—due to the rapid accumulation of fluid or toxins in the lungs and body. This happens when fluid and plasma move out of the bloodstream and into the air sacs in the lungs, interfering with the exchange of oxygen. ARDS has very diverse causes, among them pneumonia, aspiration of foreign matter (vomit, food, etc.) into the lungs, major physical trauma, severe infection, and pancreatitis.

ACUTE RESPIRATORY FAILURE (ARF) Inability of the lungs to perform their basic task: gas exchange. Lungs transfer oxygen from inhaled air into the blood, and carbon dioxide from the blood into exhaled air. Many different medical conditions can lead to respiratory failure.

AD LIB As desired.

ADENOVIRUS A group of viruses responsible for respiratory diseases (common cold, pneumonia, croup, bronchiolitis, and bronchitis), infections of the stomach and intestine (gastroenteritis), eyes (conjunctivitis), bladder (cystitis), and rashes. Patients with compromised immune systems are especially susceptible to severe complications of adenovirus infection.

ADHESION 1. The union of two opposing tissue surfaces (often in reference to the sides of a wound). 2. Scar tissue strands that form in the area of a previous operation, frequently after abdominal surgery.

ADL Activities of daily living.

ADMINISTRATION In hospital care, the act of giving (administering) a medication. The route of administration is oral or intravenous (by injection or IV line).

ADVERSE EVENT 1. In pharmacology, any unexpected or dangerous reaction to a drug. 2. In many hospitals, more broadly a surgical or medical error.

AEROSOL A fine mist or spray that contains tiny particles. A nebulizer can aerosolize a medication to be inhaled as a form of treatment.

AGAINST MEDICAL ADVICE (AMA) A term used about a patient who leaves the hospital against the advice of health-care providers; more formally, a legal term releasing a doctor and a hospital from liability if a patient leaves the hospital against a doctor's advice.

AIDS Acquired immune deficiency syndrome, the disease of the immune system that results from infection by the AIDS virus (HIV).

AIRWAY OBSTRUCTION Partial or complete blockage of the bronchial tubes, or bronchi (breathing tubes from the trachea to the lungs) due to foreign objects, allergic reactions, infections, and injury, among other causes.

ALLERGY A reaction by the body's system of defense triggered by foreign invaders, or allergens (pollens, dust mites, molds, dander, certain foods, infections), that are usually otherwise harmless.

ALLEVIATE To make easier to endure. The term is typically used in hospitals to report relief from pain or discomfort or from the symptoms associated with either.

ALOPECIA Significant hair loss, often a side effect of severe illness.

AMA Against medical advice.

AMBU BAG AND MASK A medical device consisting of a face mask attached to a rubber bag, which, when squeezed by hand, fills the lungs with oxygen and assists breathing.

AMT Amount.

ANALGESIA Inability to feel pain while still conscious.

ANALGESIC A medication that relieves pain.

ANC Absolute neutrophil count, representing the total number of white blood cells in the body that are capable of fighting bacterial infections.

ANEMIA The condition of having less than the normal number of red blood cells or less than the normal quantity of hemoglobin in the blood, a lack that decreases the oxygen-carrying capacity of the blood.

ANESTHETIC Medication administered for the relief of pain and loss of sensation during surgery. A *local or regional anesthetic* causes loss of feeling in a specific part of the body. A *general anesthetic* causes loss of awareness.

ANGINA Pain experienced in the chest area when the heart is deprived of oxygen.

ANOXIA A severe lack of oxygen going to the body and brain.

ANS Autonomic nervous system.

ANTIBIOTICS Drugs used in treating infections that either destroy harmful microorganisms (bacteria, viruses, and fungi) or slow their growth.

ANTIBODIES Protein substances in the bloodstream that are produced by the body in response to invaders, including harmful bacteria and viruses that trigger the body's defense system. Antibodies attach to the invaders, causing them to be destroyed by other cells in the immune system. Antibodies, also called immunoglobulins, are classified into five major types. *See also* immunoglobulin.

ANTICOAGULANT Any agent used to prevent the formation of blood clots.

ANTICONVULSANT A medication used to control or prevent seizures (convulsions) or stop an ongoing series of seizures.

ANTIDOTE A drug that counteracts the effect of a poison or the overdose of another drug.

ANTIGEN A chemical recognized by the body's immune system as being foreign, which triggers the formation of antibodies.

ANTIMICROBIALS Antibiotics, antivirals, or antifungals.

ANTIREFLUX SURGERY (FUNDOPLICATION) A surgical technique that strengthens the barrier against acid reflux (acid coming back up from the stomach) when the lower esophageal sphincter does not work normally.

ANXIETY An unpleasant state that involves a complex combination of emotions, including fear, apprehension, and worry, often accompanied by such physical sensations as heart palpitations, nausea, chest pain, shortness of breath, and tension headache.

APLASIA *See* hypoplasia.

APNEA *See* sleep apnea.

APPENDECTOMY Surgical removal of the appendix to treat acute appendicitis.

APPENDICITIS Inflammation of the appendix due to infection, requiring, in acute cases, the removal of the appendix (appendectomy).

ARDS Acute respiratory distress syndrome.

ARF Acute respiratory failure.

ARRHYTHMIA Any deviation from the normal pattern of the heartbeat; a heartbeat that is too fast or too slow or irregular in its pattern.

ARTERIAL CATHETER (A-LINE, INTRA-ARTERIAL CATHETER) A special catheter that is placed in an artery and used to check blood pressure and draw blood samples.

ARTIFICIAL VENTILATION Use of manual or mechanical means to support breathing when normal breathing is inefficient or has stopped.

ASAP As soon as possible.

ASD Atrial septal defect.

ASPIRATION 1. Taking solid or liquid material into the lung passages. 2. A procedure done by a doctor to remove fluids or materials by inserting a needle or a tube into an abscess or lump.

ASSESSMENT A periodic physical examination by a doctor, nurse, respiratory therapist, or other health-care professional.

ASSISTIVE DEVICE Any device designed, made, and/or adapted to assist a person to perform a particular task or tasks. Examples are canes, crutches, walkers, wheelchairs, and shower chairs.

ASTHMA A common disorder in which chronic inflammation of the bronchial tubes, or bronchi, makes them swell, narrowing these airways to the lungs and making it difficult to breathe. Asthma involves only the bronchial tubes and does not affect the air sacs or the lung tissue itself. Airway narrowing in asthma is due to three major processes acting on the bronchi: inflammation, spasm (bronchospasm), and hyperactivity (overreaction or allergy to some substance)

ATELECTASIS Partial or complete collapse of a previously expanded lung due to loss of air in air sacs. *See also* pneumothorax.

ATRIAL SEPTAL DEFECT (ASD) A congenital defect in the heart between the atria.

ATTENDING DOCTOR The staff doctor with primary responsibility for a patient's care while the patient is in the hospital.

AUTONOMIC NERVOUS SYSTEM (ANS) The part of the nervous system that regulates involuntary function, including the heart rate, the glands, and the smooth muscles in the respiratory and digestive systems. *See also* somatic nervous system.

BASELINE The starting point for health-care providers: once a patient's illness or injury is thoroughly assessed, providers can refer back to the baseline to monitor changes or improvement.

BATHROOM PRIVILEGES (BRP) An order written by a doctor to indicate that a patient may safely, without endangering the patient's medical condition, get out of bed to use the bathroom.

BENIGN Not cancerous or malignant. A benign tumor doesn't invade surrounding tissue or spread to other parts of the body; it may grow, but it stays in the same place. Any disorder or condition that does not produce harmful effects can also be described as benign.

BETADINE A brown iodine-based liquid that kills surface bacteria when applied to the skin.

BID Twice a day. (Latin: *bis in die*)

BILIRUBIN ("BILI") A substance produced when the liver breaks down old red blood cells, which contain hemoglobin (the protein in red blood cells that carries oxygen). Bilirubin is usually removed from the body in bile, which is then eliminated through the digestive tract. When bilirubin builds up, the skin and the eyes appear yellow, a condition called jaundice.

BIOPSY Diagnostic test involving the removal of tissue or cells for examination under a microscope.

BISPECTRAL INDEX (BIS) MONITOR A device that analyzes the patient's brain wave pattern and converts it into a "depth of sedation" number so the anesthetist can continuously monitor brain function during surgery.

BLOOD CLOT Blood that has converted from a liquid to a solid state. A blood clot is potentially dangerous if it is stationary within a blood vessel (thrombus), blocking blood flow, or if it moves from that location through the bloodstream (embolus).

BLOOD GASES A blood gas test to determine the amount of oxygen and carbon dioxide in the blood and its acid-base balance (pH).

BLOOD POISONING *See* sepsis.

BLOOD PRESSURE (BP) The pressure exerted on the walls of the blood vessels by blood circulating through the body each time the heart beats. Blood pressure normally varies greatly, depending on factors like activity and mood. *See also* diastolic blood pressure; hypertension; hypotension; systolic blood pressure.

BLOOD TYPE One of the classifications (A, B, AB, or O; Rh plus or minus; etc.) into which the blood of each person can be separated based on antigens in the blood cells. Before a scheduled blood transfusion, samples from the donor and the recipient are tested to make sure they are compatible.

BLOOD UREA NITROGEN (BUN) TEST A test to measure the amount of nitrogen in the blood in the form of urea, a waste product formed when the body breaks down protein and which is eliminated from the bloodstream by the kidneys.

BLUE BLOOD (VENOUS BLOOD) Blood in the veins of the body that is returning to the heart, where it will be pumped to the lungs to pick up oxygen (becoming red blood) and circulate through the body again. *See also* red blood.

BLUNT ABDOMINAL INJURY Injury to the abdomen caused by something that struck that area of the body but did not penetrate the skin.

BM Bowel movement.

BOLUS Administration of fluid or medication in a large single dose, given to raise blood concentration to an effective level. A bolus is also used in radiation therapy to fill in irregular body surfaces in order to assure the targeted treatment.

BONE MARROW A spongy material found in the center of the bone containing stem cells that manufacture blood cells. The three major types of blood cells produced are red blood cells (RBCs), white blood cells (WBCs), and platelets.

BONE MARROW BIOPSY The removal of a sample of bone marrow and a small amount of bone (usually from the hip) through a large needle. At least two samples are taken, the first by aspiration (suction with a syringe) and the second by a core biopsy to obtain bone marrow together with bone fibers. After the needle is removed, this solid sample is pushed out of the needle with a wire. Both samples are examined under a microscope to look for diseases and abnormalities and to secure a blood cell count.

BONE SCAN A technique to create images of bones on a computer screen or on film by injecting a small amount of radioactive material into the bloodstream and recording where it collects in the bones—it tends especially to collect in abnormal areas.

BORDERLINE Uncertain, indeterminate, or debatable but meriting watchful attention because the condition it describes could change—for example, borderline diabetes.

BOWEL RESECTION Surgery to remove part of the small or large intestine in order to treat various intestinal disorders, including cancer and inflammatory bowel disease, or to remove an obstruction or repair damage caused by an injury.

BOWEL SOUNDS The gurgling, rumbling, or growling noises from the abdomen caused by peristalsis (the muscle contractions that move the contents of the stomach and intestines downward). Bowel sounds are normal, but if they increase significantly in volume, a bowel obstruction of some kind could be indicated.

BP Blood pressure.

BRADYCARDIA A slow heartbeat.

BRAIN STEM The stemlike part of the brain that is connected to the spinal cord. It is the extension of the spinal cord up into the brain. The brain stem is small but important. It manages messages going between the brain and the rest of the body, and it controls basic body functions such as breathing and swallowing and manages heart rate and blood pressure.

BROVIAC OR HICKMAN CATHETER A long thin tube made of flexible silicone rubber that is surgically inserted into one of the main blood vessels leading to the heart. The catheter can be used for drawing blood samples and for giving intravenous fluids, blood, medication, or nutrition. It is often inserted to improve nutrition and monitor heart function or for long-term treatments. It may decrease the number of needles (helping to avoid needlestick) required to draw blood and is often used when IVs are not otherwise available.

BRP Bathroom privileges.

BUN TEST Blood urea nitrogen test.

BYPASS *See* heart bypass.

CA Cancer.

CAL Calories.

CANCER Diseases characterized by the uncontrolled and abnormal growth of cells.

CANDIDA A fungal infection affecting the mouth that can be very serious if the infection spreads to the blood or other body tissues.

CANNULA A slender tube that can be inserted into a body cavity or duct or placed on the outside of the nose to deliver oxygen through small prongs.

CAPILLARIES The smallest blood vessels, which distribute oxygenated blood from the arteries to the tissues of the body and gather deoxygenated blood from the tissues back into the veins. When pink areas of skin such as the fingertips are compressed, this causes blanching because blood is pressed out of the capillaries.

CAPS Capsules.

CARBON DIOXIDE (CO_2) A waste product formed by the production of energy in the cells and either eliminated by the lungs or neutralized by the kidneys.

CARDIAC ARREST The cessation of effective pumping action by the heart—most commonly due to myocardial infarction—bringing abrupt loss of consciousness, absence of the pulse, and a cessation of breathing. Unless it is treated promptly, irreversible brain damage and death can follow within minutes. *See also* heart bypass.

CARDIAC CONTUSION A bruise of the heart resulting when a person is hit in the chest or suffers a chest injury.

CARDIOMYOPATHY Weakness of the heart muscle.

CARDIOPULMONARY RESUSCITATION (CPR, "RESUS") A technique used to temporarily restore circulation and breathing to a person who has stopped breathing and whose heart has stopped beating, typically deployed with speed and under emergency conditions.

CARDIOVASCULAR SYSTEM The body's circulatory system, consisting of the heart and blood vessels, which transports nutrients (like sugar) and oxygen to the tissues and cells and removes waste products. The system moves the blood through the heart, arteries, veins, and capillaries. *See also* red blood; blue blood.

CARRIER A person who harbors the microorganisms causing a particular disease without experiencing signs or symptoms of infection and who can transmit the disease to others.

CAT SCAN *See* computed (axial) tomography.

CATH Catheterization.

CATHETER A thin flexible tube placed in a blood vessel, body opening, or cavity to drain fluid from or inject fluid into the body. The most common catheter is the Foley catheter, used to drain urine from the bladder.

CBC Complete blood count.

CC Chief complaint.

CC Cubic centimeters.

CENTIGRADE Thermometer scale in which the freezing point of water is 0 degrees and the boiling point of water at sea level is 100 degrees. The centigrade or Celsius scale is used in most of the world; the Fahrenheit scale is still commonly used in the United States. This difference requires conversion from centigrade (C) to Fahrenheit (F) degrees, and vice versa. "Normal" body temperature is 37 degrees centigrade or 98.6 degrees Fahrenheit.

If you have Fahrenheit degrees and want centigrade degrees: Subtract 32, multiply the result by 5, and divide by 9.

If you have centigrade degrees and want Fahrenheit degrees: Multiply by 9, divide the result by 5, and add 32.

CENTRAL LINE A long flexible tube inserted into a vein, usually near the elbow, and threaded up the vein until its tip reaches one of the large veins near the heart. It is typically specified for patients who need to receive fluids or medications intravenously for a long period of time. Also called a percutaneously inserted central catheter (PICC).

CENTRAL VENOUS CATHETER (CVC) *See* central venous line.

CENTRAL VENOUS LINE (CVL) A catheter with one or more tubes that are placed under the skin and directed into a large blood vessel leading into the heart, allowing fluids, medications, pressure measurements, nutrition, and blood products to be taken and given and blood to be drawn for laboratory tests, thus avoiding needlestick. Also called a central venous catheter (CVC).

CENTRAL VENOUS PRESSURE The blood pressure in the veins leading into the heart, which indicates whether the amount of blood leaving the heart balances the amount entering the heart, among other things.

CEREBRAL EDEMA A swelling of the brain due to an increase in fluids in the brain tissue, most often caused by trauma, infection, salt or sugar imbalance, shock, or anoxia.

CEREBROSPINAL FLUID (CSF) The clear, colorless fluid that surrounds the brain and spinal cord with nutrients.

CEREBROVASCULAR ACCIDENT (CVA) OR STROKE Sudden loss or impairment of brain functions that occurs when a blood vessel that supplies the brain bursts or is blocked by a clot, which causes damage or death to nerve cells in the area.

CERVICAL SPINE (C-SPINE) The seven bones (vertebrae) that make up the neck.

CF Cystic fibrosis.

CHEMOTHERAPY ("CHEMO") Drugs primarily administered to destroy cancer cells.

CHEST PHYSICAL THERAPY (CPT) A therapy involving clapping or vibrating the chest wall to loosen secretions, making them easier to cough up.

CHEST TUBES Tubes inserted through the skin into the space around the lungs to drain fluid or air.

CHEST X-RAY An X-ray picture of the chest showing the heart and lungs, any tubes or catheters located there, and possibly other things— for example, a bullet.

CHIEF COMPLAINT The primary reason for a patient's visit to the hospital; the medical condition of record.

CHOLECYSTECTOMY Surgery to remove the gallbladder. In a laparoscopic cholecystectomy a laparoscope and other surgical instruments are inserted through small incisions in the abdomen. The camera on the laparoscope allows the surgeon to see the gallbladder on a television screen and remove it through the incisions.

CHRONIC ILLNESS An illness that persists for a long period of time with very slow (if any) change.

CHRONIC OBSTRUCTIVE PULMONARY DISEASE (COPD) A disease of the lungs in which the airways become narrowed, causing shortness of breath.

CIRCULATORY SYSTEM *See* cardiovascular system.

CLOSED HEAD INJURY An injury to the brain caused by a blow to the head that does not penetrate the skull or brain tissue or by a severe shaking that can cause tearing, shearing, or stretching of the nerves at the base of the brain, blood clots, edema, and even death.

***CLOSTRIDIUM DIFFICILE* (*C. DIFFICILE,* "C-DIFF ")** The bacterium that causes an infection whose symptoms are severe diarrhea, abdominal pain, and dehydration. The infection is typically found in hospitals with less than ideal hygiene practices.

C/O Complains of.

CO$_2$ Carbon dioxide.

COAGULATION Blood clotting at the site of an injury.

COLECTOMY Surgery to remove all or part of the colon, primarily to treat colon cancer.

COLONOSCOPY A test that allows a doctor to examine the interior of the large intestine (rectum and colon) using a long flexible tube with a light and camera lens at the end (colonoscope).

COLOSTOMY A surgical operation in which an obstructed section of the colon is brought through the abdominal wall and opened in order to drain or decompress it.

COLPOSCOPY Visual examination of the cervix and vagina using a lighted magnifying instrument (colposcope).

COMA A condition in which a person is unable to respond to voice, touch, or pain. The person may move, but this is usually an involuntary response. Comas may be caused by head traumas, diseases such as diabetes, poisoning, etc.—or they may be medically induced to perform certain procedures.

COMPLETE BLOOD COUNT (CBC) A test that measures the level of hemoglobin (oxygen-carrying capacity) and the numbers of red and white blood cells and platelets in the blood.

COMPUTED (AXIAL) TOMOGRAPHY (CT SCAN, CAT SCAN) A diagnostic imaging procedure that uses a combination of X-rays and computer technology to produce cross-sectional images (often called slices), both horizontal and vertical, of the body. A CT/CAT scan shows detailed images of any part of the body, including bones, muscles, fat, and organs. CT/CAT scans are more detailed than general X-rays.

CONCERNING A term often used informally by health-care providers to describe test results, reactions, and other conditions that are not alarming but that may require watchful, ongoing attention—in essence, a heads-up for staff as well as families.

CONCUSSION The mildest and most common form of head injury, associated with a temporary loss of consciousness without other obvious injury.

CONGENITAL Existing at birth or dating from birth; hereditary.

CONGENITAL HEART DISEASE A disease present at birth caused by a structural abnormality that occurs as the heart is forming which results in an abnormal flow of blood through the heart and/or lungs.

CONSULT A shortened form of consultation used casually to refer to a request for the opinion of a specialist about a patient's condition.

CONTAGIOUS Originally used to describe a disease transmitted only by direct physical contact but now generally understood to mean any disease that can be transmitted (by coughing, etc.) from one person to another.

CONTUSION A bruise. A contusion is caused when blood vessels are damaged or broken as the result of a bump or hit to the skin. The raised area of a bump or bruise is the result of blood leaking from these injured blood vessels into the tissues, as well as the body's response to the injury. A purplish, flat bruise that occurs when blood leaks into the top layers of skin is an ecchymosis.

COPD Chronic obstructive pulmonary disease.

CPAP Continuous positive airway pressure.

CPT Chest physical therapy.

CRACKLES A sound heard in the lungs when fluid is present.

CRANIOTOMY Excision of a part of the skull; surgical opening of the skull to gain access to intracranial structures.

CRASH Cardiac arrest, in hospital jargon.

CRASH CART A trolley with the equipment and drugs needed to assist a patient who suffered cardiac arrest.

CREATININE A compound that the body synthesizes and utilizes to store energy. It is produced in the body by creatine, which is sold as a dietary supplement and used by athletes to increase muscle bulk.

CROSS-MATCHING A process to ensure that the blood between donor and recipient matches.

CSF Cerebrospinal fluid.

CT SCAN *See* computed (axial) tomography.

CULTURE A laboratory procedure in which suspect samples of blood, urine, or other body fluid are collected, and any bacteria, virus, or fungus present is encouraged to grow so that the cause of an infection can be identified before treatment.

CVA Cerebrovascular accident. Also known as a stroke.

CVC Central venous catheter. Also called a central venous line.

CVL Central venous line. Also called a central venous catheter.

CVP Central venous pressure.

CVVHD AND CAVHD (CONTINUOUS VENO-VENOUS HEMODIAFIL-TRATION AND CONTINUOUS ARTERIO-VENOUS HEMODIAFILTRA-TION) Forms of dialysis used in an ICU or operating room in which large catheters placed into veins and/or arteries allow blood to be filtered outside the body through an "artificial kidney." This machine runs continuously and requires cooperative or sedated patients.

CXR Chest X-ray.

CYANOSIS A condition in which there is not enough oxygen in the blood, causing the skin, mouth, tongue, and/or nails to look blue.

CYSTIC FIBROSIS (CF) An inherited disease in which the mucus lining the surfaces of internal organs becomes thick, dry, and sticky, affecting the functioning of the respiratory system, the sweat glands, and the digestive and reproductive systems.

CYSTOSCOPY Use of a viewing tube inserted up the urethra to examine the urethra and the bladder cavity.

DA, DAW Dispense as written.

DEBRIDEMENT Surgical removal of foreign material or dead, damaged, or infected tissue from a wound or burn.

DEEP VEIN THROMBOSIS Blood clot that occurs within deep-lying veins.

DEFIBRILLATOR An electrical device with two paddles that are placed on the chest to discharge electricity through the heart when a lethal rhythm is evident. The aim is to shock the heart rhythm back to normal. The most common lethal rhythms present during a cardiac arrest are these:

> *Asystole*—The heart has stopped beating.

> *Bradycardia*—The heart is beating so slowly that not enough blood is pumped out of it.

> *Pulseless electrical activity (PEA)*—The heart rhythm should be producing a pulse, but it isn't.

> *Ventricular fibrillation*—The ventricle (main chamber of the heart) is twitching, causing a rapid, unsynchronized, and uncoordinated heartbeat.

DEFICIT Less than normal. A term used to describe diminished cognitive or physical function due to illness or injury. Also used to describe a lack of essential vitamins or minerals.

DEHYDRATION Excessive loss of body water. Diseases of the gastrointestinal tract that cause vomiting or diarrhea may lead to dehydration.

Other causes include heat exposure, prolonged vigorous exercise (as in a marathon), kidney disease, and medications (diuretics).

DEPRESSION An illness that involves the body, mood, and thoughts, affecting the way a person eats and sleeps, the way the person feels about himself or herself, and the way the person thinks about things. Not uncommon among hospital patients with severe and prolonged conditions.

DERMATITIS Inflammation of the skin due either to direct contact with an irritating substance or to an allergic reaction. Symptoms include redness, itching, and sometimes blistering.

DIABETES A disease that develops when the pancreas does not produce enough insulin, which assists sugar (glucose) to enter cells, where it can be converted to energy.

DIALYSIS An artificial process that performs some of the functions of a normal kidney when a person's own kidneys are absent or not working properly. *Peritoneal dialysis,* the exchange of fluids through a catheter placed into the abdomen, can be performed at home. *Hemodialysis,* which requires a machine and a catheter placed into a large vein close to the heart or a large shunt placed surgically, occurs intermittently (perhaps three times a week) for approximately two to four hours each time. *See also* CVVHD and CAVHD.

DIASTOLIC BLOOD PRESSURE Blood pressure at its lowest point, when the heart is in a period of relaxation between beats. In a blood pressure reading, the diastolic pressure is the second number recorded—the 80 in a typical reading for an adult: 120/80.

DIATHERMY Use of high frequency electrical currents to generate moderate heat for therapeutic purposes and also to cauterize blood vessels during surgery to prevent excess bleeding.

DIFFERENTIAL DIAGNOSIS The complex process of comparing and contrasting two or more diseases with similar symptoms and test results in order to determine which is causing the patient's illness. The result of a differential diagnosis is a conditional or tentative diagnosis, which usually requires further testing or assessment for confirmation.

DIGESTIVE SYSTEM The organs responsible for processing food into the body and food waste out of the body and for making use of food to keep the body healthy. These organs include the salivary glands, mouth, esophagus, stomach, liver, gallbladder, pancreas, small intestine, colon, anus, and rectum.

DILATED CARDIOMYOPATHY A condition in which the heart becomes enlarged and weak, sometimes because of a virus.

DILATION AND CURETTAGE (D & C) A common gynecological surgery in which the cervical canal is widened with a dilator and the uterine cavity is scraped with a curette.

DISCHARGE 1. A patient's release from the hospital. 2. A secretion from the body, such as mucus or pus.

DIURETIC A medication that helps the kidneys pass more water, thus reducing excess fluid in the organs, especially the lungs and heart.

DNR Do not resuscitate.

DOB Date of birth.

DONOR Family member or unrelated volunteer who donates tissues, organs, or blood to a patient in need.

DOPPLER ULTRASOUND A form of ultrasound that can detect and measure blood flow.

DRESSING The covering applied to a wound to prevent infection— anything from a simple bandage to a complex series of medicated layers, chosen according to the severity and depth of the wound.

DRSG Dressing.

DRUG INTERACTION The effects of two or more medications taken together, possibly producing a reaction that is dangerous or even life-threatening.

DYSPHAGIA A condition in which swallowing is either difficult or painful to perform or in which swallowed material seems to be stalled in its passage to the stomach.

E. COLI (*ESCHERICHIA COLI*) A bacterium that normally resides in the human colon, most strains of which are quite harmless but some strains of which are capable of causing very serious diseases or even death.

ECCHYMOSIS Bruise on the skin or in mucous membranes (for example, in the intestine or mouth) caused by the escape of blood into the tissues from ruptured blood vessels.

ECG Electrocardiogram.

ECHOCARDIOGRAM (ECHO) A type of ultrasound test in which sound waves are sent through a device called a transducer and are reflected off the structures of the heart. These "echoes" are converted into pictures that can be seen on a video monitor.

ED Emergency department.

EDEMA The swelling of soft tissues as a result of excess fluid accumulation.

EEG Electroencephalogram.

EKG Electrocardiogram.

ELECTROCARDIOGRAM (ECG, EKG) A test that records the electrical activity of the heart, shows abnormal rhythms (arrhythmias or dysrhythmias), and detects heart muscle damage. Electrode patches are placed on the chest, and a machine records the electrical measurements detected that way by making a graph on a moving strip of paper.

ELECTROCOAGULATION Electrosurgery that helps harden tissue.

ELECTRODESICCATION Electrosurgery that destroys tissue.

ELECTROENCEPHALOGRAM (EEG) A test that measures and records the electrical currents within the brain, done by attaching electrode wires to the scalp and connecting them to a machine that plots the electrical impulses on paper or a computer screen.

EMBOLISM The obstruction of a blood vessel by a foreign substance or by a blood clot. Blood clots that lodge in the brain can cause strokes; those that lodge in the heart, a heart attack.

EMERGENCY ROOM, EMERGENCY DEPARTMENT (ER, ED) The department of a hospital responsible for providing emergency medical or surgical care.

EMESIS Vomiting, throwing up.

ENCEPHALITIS Inflammation of the brain caused by an infection. Treatment must begin as early as possible to avoid potentially serious and lifelong effects. Antibiotics, anti-viral medications, and anti-inflammatory drugs can all be used, depending on the cause. If brain damage results from encephalitis, therapy (such as physical therapy) may help patients regain lost functions.

ENDARTERECTOMY Surgical removal of the lining of a major artery in order to clear it of accumulated plaque.

ENDOCARDITIS An infection of the lining of the heart.

ENDOSCOPY A test that uses a small flexible tube with a light and a camera lens at the end (endoscope) to examine the inside of the digestive tract. Tissue samples may also be taken for examination and testing. In general, an endoscope is placed into the body through a natural opening like the mouth or the anus. The most common endoscopic procedures evaluate the esophagus (swallowing tube), stomach, and portions of the intestine, colon (colonoscopy), or airway (bronchoscopy).

ENDOTRACHEAL TUBE (ET TUBE) A tube inserted through the nose or mouth into the trachea (windpipe) to maintain an open airway and permit removal of secretions. This tube is usually connected to either a ventilator or a suctioning machine.

ENT Ear, nose and throat.

EPIDURAL ANESTHETIC An anesthetic that is injected into the epidural space in the middle and lower back, just outside the spinal space, to numb the lower extremities.

EPILEPSY *See* seizure disorder.

EPISODE *See* event.

ER Emergency room.

ERYTHEMA Redness of the skin resulting from inflammation—for example, sunburn.

ERYTHROCYTES Red blood cells.

ESOPHAGUS The muscular canal that runs from the larynx (voice box) to the stomach.

ET TUBE Endotracheal tube.

ETA Estimated time of arrival.

ETIOLOGY The study of causes, mainly in medicine. It refers to attempts to discover the cause or origin of disease and the factors that produce it. In medical-speak, "the etiology is unknown" translates as "we don't know the cause."

EVENT A term often used interchangeably with *episode* to describe a seizure or other occurrence with implications that are typically unpleasant. *See also* adverse event.

EXANTHEMA A rash caused by harmful bacteria, a virus, or an illness.

EXPOSURE Contact with someone with a contagious disease, potentially causing the exposed person to contract the disease.

EXSANGUINATE To drain of blood; to bleed to death.

EXTUBATE To remove a tube from a hollow organ or passageway, typically the airway. The opposite of extubate is intubate.

FAHRENHEIT Thermometer scale in which the freezing point of water is 32 degrees and the boiling point of water 212 degrees. Most hospitals, even in the United States, use the centigrade scale instead. For a formula to convert from centigrade to Fahrenheit, *see* centigrade.

FALLOPIAN TUBES Tubes that extend from the uterus to the ovaries and transport eggs and sperm.

FASTING BLOOD SUGAR A method for learning how much glucose (sugar) there is in a blood sample taken after a period of time without eating or drinking anything. It is usually performed prior to breakfast.

FEBRILE Feverish or having a temperature. *See also* fever.

FEBRILE SEIZURE A convulsion (seizure) that occurs in association with a rapid increase in body temperature.

FECAL Relating to the feces, stool.

FELLOW A doctor who has completed residency and who is undertaking further specialty training.

FEVER A higher than normal body temperature. Although a fever is technically any body temperature above 98.6 degrees Fahrenheit (37 degrees centigrade), in practice a person is usually not considered to have a significant fever until the temperature is above 100.4 degrees Fahrenheit (38 degrees centigrade).

FIBRILLATION Rapid and chaotic beating of the many individual muscle fibers of the heart, which is consequently unable to maintain effective synchronous contraction. The affected part of the heart then ceases to pump blood.

FIBRIN SEALANTS A new class of sealants, made from plasma, that help to stop oozing from small blood vessels during surgery when conventional surgical techniques are not feasible. The sealants, which form a flexible shield over the oozing blood vessel, help control bleeding within minutes.

FLAT-LINED An informal clinical term to confirm that a patient's heart has stopped, as evidenced by the flat line displayed on a heart monitor.

FLATUS Gas in the intestinal tract or passed through the anus. The intestinal gases are hydrogen, nitrogen, carbon dioxide, and methane, all of which are odorless. The unpleasant smell of flatus is the result of trace gases such as indole, skatole, and, most commonly, hydrogen sulfide. When people fart, they are passing flatus.

FLU (INFLUENZA) A disease that can be caused by viruses of many types—designated A, B, C, etc.—that infect the respiratory tract. Most people who get the flu recover completely in one to two weeks, but some people develop serious and potentially life-threatening medical complications, such as pneumonia.

FOLEY CATHETER A thin plastic tube placed in the bladder to drain urine.

FRACTURE A break in the bone or cartilage, usually a result of trauma.

FREE SKIN GRAFT Surgery in which healthy skin is detached from one part of the body to repair areas of lost or damaged skin in another part of the body.

G, GM Gram.

GAIT The way a person walks. Important for medical assessment, when an "unsteady gait" can be cause for concern.

GASTRECTOMY Partial (subtotal) or complete (total) removal of the stomach.

GASTROENTERITIS Inflammation of the stomach and the intestines, which is caused by infectious microorganisms (viruses, bacteria, etc.), food poisoning, or physical or emotional stress and which can induce nausea, vomiting, and diarrhea.

GASTROESOPHAGEAL REFLUX DISEASE (GERD) A disease involving the return of the stomach contents back up into the esophagus. Reflux frequently causes heartburn, because of irritation to the esophagus by the stomach acid, and may cause aspiration and pneumonia. Reflux becomes a disease when it is chronic and severe.

GASTROINTESTINAL (GI) Pertaining to the digestive tract, which includes the mouth, throat, esophagus, stomach, small and large intestine, anus, and rectum.

GASTROSTOMY A surgical opening into the stomach, usually made to insert a feeding tube (gastrostomy tube) and usually done to deliver nutrition directly to the stomach for patients who can't swallow. *See also* percutaneous endoscopic gastrostomy.

GB Gallbladder.

GENERAL ANESTHETIC An anesthetic that causes the patient to become unconscious, used during surgery.

GENERIC NAME (OF A DRUG) 1. The chemical name of a drug. 2. The chemical composition of a drug as opposed to the advertised brand name. 3. The name under which a drug is marketed (its chemical name) without advertising. Generic drugs are less expensive than brand-name drugs, but they are chemically identical and meet U.S. and Canadian standards for safety, purity, and effectiveness.

GENETICS The scientific study of heredity and genes.

GI Gastrointestinal.

GLAND 1. A group of cells that secrete a substance for use in the body—for example, the thyroid gland, which produces hormones to regulate body functions. 2. A group of cells that collect materials from the circulatory system—for example, lymph glands, which collect and neutralize bacteria and abnormal cells, which is why they swell when someone has a sore throat.

GLUCOSE (FORMERLY DEXTROSE) The chief source of energy for the body's living cells. As the main sugar that the body manufactures, glucose is generated from all three elements of food (protein, fat, and carbohydrates), but in largest part from carbohydrates. It is carried to each cell through the bloodstream.

GRAND ROUNDS A term that originally referred to an educational opportunity for doctors to meet and discuss one or more interesting patient cases but now often refers to any in-hospital educational event that might be of interest to health-care providers generally.

GRANULATION TISSUE Rough, pink tissue containing capillaries that forms around the edges of a wound. Granulation of a wound is normal and desirable.

GRANULOCYTE A type of white blood cell that helps fight infections.

GTT Drops.

G-TUBE Gastrostomy tube.

H Hour.

H & P (Medical) history and physical (examination).

H/A Headache.

H$_2$O Water.

HCT Hematocrit.

HEART ATTACK *See* myocardial infarction.

HEART BYPASS, CARDIAC BYPASS Surgery in which narrowed or blocked coronary arteries are circumvented ("bypassed") by grafting in blood vessels from elsewhere in the body to allow blood circulation to the heart.

HEART MURMUR A sound made by blood flowing through the heart, not considered alarming but sometimes caused by a heart defect.

HEART RATE The rate at which the heart beats, normally between 60 and 100 beats per minute for an adult.

HEMATOCRIT (HCT) A measurement of the percentage of space that red blood cells take up in the blood—more precisely, the proportion of the blood that consists of packed red blood cells, expressed as a percentage by volume. A normal hematocrit is between 32 and 60 percent, depending on sex, age, and health status. A low hematocrit could indicate anemia.

HEMATOMA An abnormal localized collection of clotted or partially clotted blood, usually within an organ or a soft tissue space—for example, within a muscle—caused by a break in the wall of a blood vessel. The break may be spontaneous, as in the case of an aneurysm, or caused by trauma.

HEMOCCULT, OCCULT A term for blood that is not visible to the naked eye or readily apparent. Occult blood is present in such small quantities (for example, in the feces) that it can be detected only with a microscope or by chemical testing.

HEMOGLOBIN (HGB) The oxygen-carrying protein pigment in red blood cells. Hemoglobin forms an unstable, reversible bond with oxygen, allowing for its easy release to cells. In its oxygenated state it is called *oxyhemoglobin* and is bright red. In its reduced or used state it is called *deoxyhemoglobin* and is purple-blue.

HEMOGLOBIN TEST A measurement of the amount of oxygen-carrying protein in the blood.

HEMORRHAGE Bleeding or blood loss, which could require transfusions to prevent shock.

HEMORRHOIDECTOMY Surgical removal of hemorrhoids.

HEMORRHOIDS Distended veins in the lining of the anus.

HEMOTHORAX A condition in which an abnormal collection of blood surrounds the lungs.

HERNIA Protrusion of an organ through an abnormal opening in the muscle wall of the cavity that surrounds it. The most common types are *inguinal* (a portion of the intestine protrudes into the groin muscles) and *hiatus* (a portion of the stomach protrudes upward through the diaphragm).

HFOV High-frequency oscillatory ventilation.

HGB Hemoglobin.

HICKMAN CATHETER *See* Broviac or Hickman catheter.

HIGH BLOOD PRESSURE *See* hypertension.

HIGH-FREQUENCY OSCILLATORY VENTILATION (HFOV) Use of very high rates (over 150 breaths per minute) and small volumes to provide oxygen to a patient with damaged lungs who needs assistance breathing. With HFOV, the ventilator supplies the oxygen at a lower pressure than it does conventionally, thus decreasing the risk of damage to the lung tissue (barotrauma) while improving oxygenation.

HISTORY AND PHYSICAL (H & P) The initial medical history and clinical physical examination of the patient. In a "focused" H & P the doctor concentrates on the problem reported by the patient.

HIV Human immunodeficiency virus, which infects and destroys cells of the immune system and causes AIDS.

H/O (Medical) history of (a patient).

HOB Head of bed.

HORMONE A chemical substance produced in the body that controls and regulates the activity of certain cells or organs. Specialized glands such as the thyroid secrete many hormones. Hormones are essential for a variety of activities, including the processes of digestion, metabolism, growth, reproduction, and mood control. Many hormones, such as the neurotransmitters, are active in more than one physical process.

HOSPICE A place for end-of-life care for patients facing a terminal illness and for whom regular hospital care no longer offers any options for recovery. The goal of hospice care is to reduce the severity of symptoms through therapies like pain management and also to provide emotional support for the patient and the family without taking extraordinary steps to prolong life.

HT Height.

HTN Hypertension.

HX (Medical) history (of a patient).

HYDROCEPHALUS An abnormal buildup of cerebrospinal fluid (CSF) in the ventricles of the brain, which often produces increased intracranial pressure (ICP) and can compress and damage the brain. Sometimes called water on the brain.

HYPERALIMENTATION ("HYPERAL") *See* total parenteral nutrition.

HYPERTENSION Blood pressure that is abnormally high for a person's age. When an adult is relaxed, the blood pressure is normally about 120/80. Minor variances should not be considered alarming. Simply put, the higher number represents the pressure while the heart is beating (systolic pressure); the lower number represents the pressure when the heart is resting between beats (diastolic pressure). People with chronic high blood pressure risk strokes and heart attacks.

HYPERTONIA Increased tightness of muscle tone; spasticity. Untreated, hypertonia can lead to loss of function and deformity. Treatment is by physical and/or occupational therapy and sometimes by muscle relaxant medication. Injections of botulinum toxin type A (Botox) are a recent treatment for chronic hypertonia in cerebral palsy and other disorders.

HYPERVENTILATE To breathe at an abnormally high rate, even when the body is at rest.

HYPOPLASIA Underdevelopment or incomplete development of a tissue or an organ—for example, hypoplasia of the enamel of the teeth.

Hypoplasia is less drastic than aplasia (where there is no development at all).

HYPOPLASTIC VENTRICLE A condition in which the right or left ventricle of the heart is small because it has not developed properly.

HYPOTENSION Any blood pressure that is below the normal rate, depending on age and other variables. Hypotension is the opposite of hypertension (high blood pressure). Minor variances shouldn't be considered alarming.

HYPOTHERMIA An abnormally low body temperature. Hypothermia becomes life-threatening below a body temperature of 32.2 degrees centigrade (90 degrees Fahrenheit).

HYPOTONIA Decreased tone of skeletal muscles; floppiness.

HYPOXIA A shortage of oxygen in the body.

HYSTERECTOMY Surgical removal of the uterus. In an *abdominal hysterectomy* the uterus is removed through the abdomen via a surgical incision. In a *total hysterectomy* the entire uterus is removed, including the cervix but not the fallopian tubes and the ovaries. In a *total hysterectomy with bilateral salpingo-oophorectomy,* the entire uterus, the fallopian tubes, and the ovaries are removed.

I & D Incision and drainage.

I & O Intake and output (of fluids).

ICU Intensive-care unit (of a hospital).

IDIOPATHIC In medicine, a disease or condition with an unknown cause.

IG Immunoglobulin.

ILEUS Partial or complete blockage of the intestine caused by paralysis of the bowel (a lack of peristalsis). The paralysis does not need to be complete to cause ileus, but the intestine must be so inactive that food cannot pass through. Ileus, usually a transient problem that causes constipation and bloating, commonly follows some types of surgery and can also result from certain drugs, injuries, and illnesses. A doctor listening to the abdomen with a stethoscope will hear no bowel sounds (because the bowel is inactive). Ileus may also be called paralytic ileus.

IM Intramuscular; into the muscle.

IMMUNE SYSTEM The body's system of defenses against disease and allergies. The immune system primarily consists of white blood cells and antibodies, but it includes other agents as well.

IMMUNOGLOBULIN (IG) Antibody. An essential part of the body's immune system, immunoglobulins attach to foreign substances, such as bacteria, and destroy them. There are five classes of immunoglobulins: A, D, E, G, and M.

IMMUNOGLOBULIN A (IGA) A class of immunoglobulins found in serum and external body secretions such as saliva, tears, and sweat, as well as in the gastrointestinal, respiratory, and genitourinary tracts.

IMMUNOGLOBULIN D (IGD) A class of immunoglobulins found on the surface of B cells (B-lymphocytes). Almost nothing is known about the normal function of these immunoglobulins.

IMMUNOGLOBULIN E (IGE) A class of immunoglobulins that includes the antibodies elicited by an allergic substance (allergen). A person who has an allergy usually has elevated blood levels of IgE. These antibodies attack the invading army of allergens.

IMMUNOGLOBULIN G (IGG) A class of immunoglobulins also known as gamma globulins that includes many of the most common antibodies circulating in the blood. Intravenous IgG is sometimes given to aid in fighting infections or immune diseases.

IMMUNOGLOBULIN M (IGM) A class of immunoglobulins that includes the antibodies produced first in an immune response and later replaced by other types of antibodies. Their presence indicates acute or recent infection.

IMMUNOSUPPRESSED, IMMUNOCOMPROMISED A term describing the body's reduced ability to fight infections because the immune system is not active or effective.

INCONTINENCE Inability to control excretions. *Urinary incontinence* is the inability to keep urine in the bladder. *Fecal incontinence* is the inability to retain feces in the rectum.

INDWELLING (CATHETER) Intended to remain within the body for a long period of time.

INFECTION Invasion of the body by harmful microorganisms that reproduce and multiply, causing disease.

INFILTRATE To cause (a fluid) to penetrate. If an IV line infiltrates, the fluid in the line filters outside the vein and permeates the surrounding tissue.

INFLAMMATION The body's basic reaction to infection, irritation, or other injury, the key features being redness, warmth, swelling, and pain. Inflammation is now recognized as a type of nonspecific immune response.

INFORMED CONSENT FORM A form signed by the patient (or designated next-of-kin or proxy) prior to surgery or any significant treatment that may involve experimental protocols or drugs. The form should clearly explain the proposed surgery or treatment, the intended results, and any potential risks to the patient, and it must be signed before the procedure is done, except in an emergency situation. Where English is not the primary language, most hospitals provide translators to explain treatments and options.

INFUSE 1. To introduce a fluid other than blood—perhaps a saline (salt) solution—into a vein for therapeutic reasons. 2. To introduce a fluid into the rectum to perform an enema.

INPATIENT SURGERY Surgery that requires the patient to be admitted to and stay in the hospital at least overnight.

INSULT A term used by health-care providers to describe any dangerous trauma endured by the body, including a major injury or critical illness.

INTAKE A term that typically refers to fluid intake—what a person either consumes orally or receives intravenously.

INTAKE AND OUTPUT (I & O) An accounting of fluid taken in either orally or intravenously, then lost or secreted.

INTENSIVIST A doctor who specializes in intensive-care medicine (also called critical-care medicine).

INTERCOSTAL SPACE The space between any two ribs.

INTERN A doctor who has completed medical school and who is at the hospital for additional on-the-job training.

INTRA-AORTIC BALLOON PUMP (IABP) A pump connected to a catheter inserted into the groin to help the heart pump blood.

INTRA-ARTERIAL Into an artery. Intra-arterial chemotherapy is administered directly into an artery or an organ.

INTRACELLULAR FLUID The fluid normally present inside each cell in the body.

INTRACRANIAL PRESSURE CATHETER (ICP) A catheter inserted into the brain to monitor brain swelling or to drain excess fluid from the brain. The procedure for inserting the tube through the skull is called a ventriculostomy.

INTRADERMAL Into the skin. With an intradermal injection the needle of a syringe is inserted into the skin to deliver a medication, as opposed to delivery into a muscle (intramuscular), just below the skin (subcutaneous), or into a vein (intravenous).

INTRAMUSCULAR (IM) Into a muscle. With an intramuscular injection, the needle of a syringe is inserted into a muscle to deliver a medication, as opposed to delivery into the skin (intradermal), just below the skin (subcutaneous), or into a vein (intravenous).

INTRAVENOUS (IV) 1. Into a vein. 2. A solution administered into a vein. 3. The device used to administer a solution into a vein. With an intravenous injection, the needle of a syringe is inserted into a vein, as opposed to into the skin (intradermal), just below the skin (subcutaneous), or into a muscle (intramuscular). Intravenous antibiotics are solutions containing antibiotics that are administered directly into a vein with a syringe or by intravenous catheter.

INTUBATE *See* extubate.

INVASIVE TEST A procedure or examination that requires that the body be entered in some way, using a needle or a tube—or a finger, in the case of a rectal examination.

IRRIGATE To wash out or flush—for example, a wound.

ISCHEMIA Inadequate blood supply to a local area (such as a wound) due to blockage of the blood vessels. *See also* transient ischemic attack.

ISOLATION Keeping a patient's exposure to and contact with others to a minimum in order to reduce the risk of infecting the patient or the risk of a patient infecting others.

ISOTONIC SOLUTION A solution with the same salt concentration as the normal cells of the body and the blood. An isotonic beverage (such as Gatorade) may be drunk to replace the fluid and minerals that the body uses during physical activity.

IV Intravenous; into a vein.

IV PUMP A machine that controls the delivery of fluids and medications through an intravenous catheter.

JAUNDICE Yellowish staining of the skin and sclera (whites of the eyes) by abnormally high levels of the bile pigment bilirubin in the bloodstream. The yellowing, which can extend to other tissues and body fluids, suggests liver or gallbladder problems.

JUGULAR Of or relating to any of several veins in the neck that drain blood from the head toward the heart. Catheters may be placed in these veins for procedures.

K Potassium.

KETOACIDOSIS A feature of uncontrolled diabetes. Ketosis is the accumulation of substances called ketone bodies in the blood. Acidosis is increased acidity of the blood. Symptoms of ketoacidosis include rapid or deep breathing with a fruity odor to the breath; confusion; frequent urination (polyuria); poor appetite; and eventually loss of consciousness. The treatment of ketoacidosis is a matter of urgency and is usually done in a hospital. It may require the administration of intravenous fluids, insulin, and glucose.

KG Kilogram.

KIDNEYS, URETER, AND BLADDER (KUB) An abdominal X-ray of the kidneys, ureter, bladder, and other structures, such as the diaphragm and the pelvis.

KUB Kidneys, ureter, and bladder.

KVO Keep vein open.

KYPHOSIS Outward curvature of the spine, causing a humped back.

LABILE Unstable, unsteady, not fixed.

LACERATION A cut or tear in the skin producing a wound with irregular edges.

LACTIC ACIDOSIS Acidosis due to the buildup of lactic acid (from glucose) when it is created faster than it can be metabolized. The signs are unusually deep and rapid breathing, vomiting, and abdominal pain. It can occur in cases of out-of-control diabetes, shock, hypoxia, or anoxia.

LACTOSE INTOLERANCE Inability to digest lactose, a component of dairy products. Lactose is sometimes used as an ingredient in nondairy foods, so those with a lactase deficiency (not enough of the enzyme required to digest lactose) need to check labels carefully. The most common symptoms of lactose intolerance are diarrhea, bloating, and gas.

LAMINECTOMY Surgery to remove a portion of the lamina (the layer of bone forming the walls of the vertebrae) in order to provide more room in the vertebral canal. Indicated for a spinal disc hernia or spinal canal stenosis.

LAPAROSCOPY Surgery in which a small incision is made in the abdominal wall through which a laparoscope, a flexible tube with a light and a camera lens at the end, is inserted to examine organs and check for abnormalities. Tubes, probes, and other instruments can be inserted through the same hole, and tissue samples can be taken. A laparoscope allows a number of surgical procedures (such as hernia re-pairs) to be performed without making large incisions. Also called key-hole or pinhole surgery.

LAPAROTOMY An operation to open the abdomen.

LARYNGOSCOPE A flexible lighted instrument inserted through the mouth or nose and used to examine the inside of the larynx (voice box).

LARYNGOSCOPY Inspection of the larynx (voice box) with a viewing tube (laryngoscope).

LAVAGE Washing out. In a gastric lavage the stomach is washed out to remove drugs or poisons.

LAXATIVE Something that loosens the bowels, prescribed to combat constipation.

LB Pound.

LEFT VENTRICULAR FAILURE A condition in which the left ventri-cle, the main pumping chamber of the heart, is weakened, stiff, or oth-erwise unable to function at full capacity. Right ventricular failure also occurs.

LESION A zone of damaged tissue whose function is impaired as a re-sult of disease or wounding. Primary lesions include wounds, ab-scesses, ulcers, and tumors. Secondary lesions (such as crusts and scars) are derived from primary ones.

LETHARGY Abnormal drowsiness; stupor.

LEUKEMIA A cancer of the bone marrow and blood that is character-ized by the abnormal growth of white blood cells.

LEUKOCYTE A type of white blood cell.

LFT Liver function test.

LICENSED PRACTICAL NURSE (LPN) A nurse who has graduated from an accredited school of vocational nursing but has less extensive clinical training than a registered nurse does.

LIVER FUNCTION TEST (LFT) Measurements from blood samples that reveal how well the liver is functioning.

LIVING WILL Written document that specifies restrictions on medical treatment in the event that a hospital patient is unable to communicate.

LOBECTOMY Surgical removal of a lobe of the lung, typically to excise a malignant tumor.

LOC Level of consciousness; loss of consciousness.

LOCAL ANESTHESIA An anesthetic injected into the site of an operation to temporarily numb that area.

LOS Length of stay.

LOWER GASTROINTESTINAL SERIES (LOWER GI SERIES) A series of X-rays of the colon and rectum taken after the patient is given a barium enema. Barium is a white, chalky substance that outlines the colon and rectum on the X-ray.

LP Lumbar puncture.

LPN Licensed practical nurse.

LUMBAR PUNCTURE (LP) A procedure to remove spinal fluid from the spinal canal for diagnostic testing. Other names for a lumbar puncture include spinal tap and spinal puncture. An LP can also be done to administer antibiotics, cancer drugs, or anesthetic agents into the spinal canal.

LUMPECTOMY Surgery to remove a tumor and small amounts of surrounding tissue, typically to confirm through laboratory tests whether the tumor is malignant.

LUNG CONTUSION A bruise in the lung caused by an injury to the chest.

LYMPH NODES Small bean-shaped organs located throughout the lymphatic system. The lymph nodes store special cells that can trap cancer cells or bacteria traveling through the body in lymph fluid. Also called lymph glands.

LYMPHADENOPATHY Abnormally enlarged lymph nodes, commonly called swollen glands.

LYMPHOCYTE One type of the small white blood cells (leukocytes) that play a large role in defending the body against disease. Lymphocytes are responsible for immune responses. There are two main types of lymphocytes: B-cells and T-cells. The B-cells make antibodies that attack bacteria and toxins; the T-cells attack body cells that have been taken over by viruses or become cancerous.

LYSIS 1. Destruction of a cell or molecule. *Hemolysis* is the destructive breakdown of red blood cells, limiting their ability to carry oxygen. *Bacteriolysis* is the destruction of bacteria. 2. Gradual reduction in the symptoms of a disease.

MAGNETIC RESONANCE IMAGING (MRI) A radiology technique using magnetism, radio waves, and a computer to produce images of internal body tissues. The MRI scanner is a tubular chamber surrounded by a giant circular magnet. The patient is placed on a moveable bed that is inserted into the chamber. A computer processes the information received, and an image is produced, often making it possible to detect tiny changes of structures within the body. The procedure is noisy and usually takes at least an hour.

MALABSORPTION Poor intestinal absorption of nutrients.

MALAISE A vague feeling of discomfort—one that cannot be pinned down. The patient often describes feeling "not right."

MALIGNANCY (OF A TUMOR) The exhibition of cancerous qualities. A malignant tumor may invade and destroy nearby tissue and may spread cancer (metastasize) to other parts of the body via the bloodstream or lymphatic system.

MARS Medication administration record sheet.

MASTECTOMY Surgery to remove part or all of one or both breasts, typically performed to remove a malignant tumor. In a *simple mastectomy,* only breast tissue is removed. In a *radical mastectomy,* the entire breast, some chest muscles, and all lymph nodes in the armpit are removed. In a *modified radical mastectomy,* the large muscles of the chest that move the arm are preserved.

MAX Maximum.

MEDICAL ADMINISTRATION RECORD SHEET (MARS) A formal record of hospital medications administered to a particular patient by date, time, and dose. It is consulted and updated daily by nurses and others responsible for administering medications.

MEDICAL STUDENTS (IN A HOSPITAL) Usually students completing their last few years of medical school who work under close supervision and do not make independent decisions about diagnoses or treatments.

MEMBRANE A thin layer of tissue surrounding the whole or part of an organ or the tissue lining a cavity or separating adjacent structures or cavities.

MENINGITIS An infection of the membranes that envelop the brain and spinal cord, usually due to a bacterial infection but sometimes caused by viruses or other agents. In some cases, the cause is unknown.

METABOLIC Relating to metabolism, the whole range of biochemical processes that occur within any living organism. Metabolism consists of anabolism (the buildup of substances) and catabolism (the breakdown of substances). The term is often used to refer specifically to the breakdown of food and its transformation into energy.

METASTATIC Spreading (of a cancer) to parts of the body distant from the original or primary site of the cancer.

METHICILLIN-RESISTANT *STAPHYLOCOCCUS AUREUS* (MRSA) A bacterium that causes dangerous infections that are resistant to certain antibiotics.

MG Milligram.

MITRAL VALVE REPLACEMENT (MVR) Heart surgery in which a patient's mitral valve is replaced by another valve, which may be mechanical. Typical causes of mitral valve damage include aging, infection, and a heart attack.

ML Milliliter.

MONITOR To keep track of; to watch over. Monitoring is an important task in hospital care, particularly for patients whose prognosis may be uncertain.

MORBID A term used to describe a negative, unhealthy state of mind.

MORBIDITY Rate of illness or disease within a given population or geographical location.

MORTALITY A fatal outcome; death.

MORTALITY RATE Death rate. Different types of mortality rates are calculated depending on the population and the illness or disease being considered.

MRI Magnetic resonance imaging.

MRSA Methicillin-resistant *Staphylococcus aureus*.

MUCOUS Pertaining to mucus, a thick fluid produced by the linings of some tissues.

MULTIPLE ORGAN DYSFUNCTION SYNDROME (MODS) A condition usually affecting critically ill patients in which various organs are functioning erratically or not at all. Often a sign that death may be imminent.

MVA Motor vehicle accident.

MVR Mitral valve replacement.

MYALGIA Pain in a muscle or multiple muscles.

MYOCARDIAL INFARCTION A sudden and severe chest pain (angina) that may spread to the arms and throat. Commonly called a heart attack.

MYOPATHY A neuromuscular disorder in which the prime symptom is muscle weakness due to the abnormal condition and function of the muscle fiber. Other symptoms can include muscle cramps, stiffness, and spasm.

MYOSITIS Inflammation of muscle tissue caused by injury, medications, and diseases, among other things.

MYRINGOTOMY A tiny surgical incision in the eardrum made to drain fluid or remove thickened secretions behind the eardrum.

N & V Nausea and vomiting.

N/A Not applicable.

NA Sodium (salt).

NAD No acute distress.

NASOGASTRIC (NG) TUBE A flexible tube made of rubber or plastic that is passed through the nose down into the stomach. It can be used to remove the contents of the stomach, including air, small solid objects, and poisonous fluids, or to deliver substances (nutrients or medications) into the stomach when a patient cannot eat by mouth.

NASOJEJUNAL (NJ) TUBE A flexible tube made of rubber or plastic that is passed through the nose into the jejunum (small bowel) to provide nutrition.

NAUSEA A general feeling of queasiness; the urge to vomit. Causes include systemic illness (such as influenza), medications, pain, and inner ear disease.

NEBULIZER A device for administering a medication by spraying a fine mist into the nose and mouth. Also known as an atomizer.

NECROSIS The death of living cells or tissues, often due to lack of blood flow.

NEEDLE BIOPSY (OF THE BREAST) Procedure to remove a small piece of breast tissue using a needle with a special cutting edge, done after using a local anesthetic.

NEEDLESTICK A dangerous accident in which a health-care provider suffers a puncture of the skin while handling sharps—needles, scalpels, and other sharp instruments.

NEG Negative.

NEONATE A newborn baby.

NEPHRECTOMY Surgical removal of the kidney.

NEURALGIA Pain along the course of a nerve.

NEUTROPENIA An insufficient quantity of neutrophils (circulating white blood cells) in the blood, which lowers the barrier to infection. May occur with viral infections or after radiation therapy and chemotherapy. Precautions like keeping flowers away from the patient, having visitors wear masks, gowns, and gloves, and placing the patient in isolation help to keep potential infections down.

NEUTROPHIL A type of white blood cell that plays a major role in fighting bacterial and fungal infections. A neutrophil has a lifespan of about three days.

NG Nasogastric.

NICU Neonatal intensive care unit (for premature babies and/or ill newborns).

NITRIC OXIDE A gas given to a patient on a ventilator to help improve the ability of oxygen to cross into the bloodstream when the lungs are infected or damaged.

NITROGLYCERIN (NITRO; NTG) A medication that promotes the dilation of blood vessels, which may ease chest pain associated with heart problems.

NJ TUBE Nasojenunal tube.

NKA No known allergies.

NKDA No known drug allergies.

NO., # Number.

NONINVASIVE TEST A procedure or examination that does not require that anything be inserted into the body.

NORMAL SINUS RHYTHM (NSR) The normal pattern of the heartbeat as measured by an electrocardiogram (ECG).

NP Nurse practitioner.

NPO Nothing by mouth; nothing to eat or drink, usually within a defined time frame (Latin: *non per os*).

N/S Normal saline (solution).

NSG Nursing.

NSR Normal sinus rhythm.

NTG Nitroglycerin.

NURSE PRACTITIONER (NP) A registered nurse with at least a master's degree in nursing and advanced education in a medical specialty.

NUTRITION The science or practice of taking in and utilizing foods or nourishing substances for cell growth, energy, and resistance to infections. Nutrition can be taken by mouth, IV line, NJ tube, or NG tube.

NWB Non-weight-bearing (said of a leg).

O$_2$ SAT (PRONOUNCED "OH-TWO SAT") Oxygen saturation.

OB Obstetrical; obstetrics.

OBESITY The state of being overweight. People have traditionally been considered obese if they are more than 20 percent over their ideal weight. That ideal weight must take into account the person's height, age, sex, and build.

OB-GYN (PRONOUNCED "O-B-G-Y-N") Obstetrics and gynecology; a doctor who specializes in obstetrics and gynecology.

OBSTRUCTIVE SLEEP APNEA *See* sleep apnea.

OBTUNDED Mentally dulled. Head trauma may obtund a person.

OCCLUDE To close, obstruct, or prevent passage. To occlude an artery is to obstruct the flow of blood.

OCCULT *See* hemoccult.

OCCUPATIONAL THERAPY (OT) Therapy to help learn or relearn the activities of daily living and developmental skills.

ODA Operating-day admission (of a patient).

OINT Ointment.

OLIGURIA Significantly decreased production of urine, typically due to dehydration, renal failure, or an obstruction in the urinary tract.

ONCOLOGY The study and treatment of cancer.

OOB Out of bed.

OPEN FRACTURE A fracture in which the bone protrudes through the skin. Also called a compound fracture.

OR Operating room.

ORDERS The course of treatment prescribed by a doctor, including any drugs or therapies.

OSTEOMYELITIS Inflammation of the bone due to infection. Osteomyelitis is sometimes a complication of surgery or injury, although infection can also reach bone tissue through the bloodstream.

OSTOMY An operation (such as a colostomy) to create an opening from an area inside the body to the outside for the purpose of waste elimination.

OT Occupational therapy.

OTC Over the counter. The term refers to medications that can be bought without a prescription.

OUTPATIENT SURGERY Surgery that does not require a hospital stay.

OUTRAGEOUS An adjective used informally to describe a test result that is not alarming: "nothing outrageous."

OXYGEN (O_2) A colorless, odorless gas found in air and required to sustain life. The percentage of oxygen typically found in room air is 21 percent. Oxygen can be given in concentrations up to 100 percent using special delivery devices such as a mask or endotracheal tube.

OXYGEN SATURATION (O_2 SAT) A measurement of the percentage of hemoglobin that is carrying oxygen. A normal oxygen saturation is about 93 percent.

OXYGENATION The amount of oxygen in the blood or other fluid.

OZ Ounce.

P Pulse.

PA Physician assistant.

PAC Premature atrial contraction.

PACEMAKER A small battery-driven device usually placed under the skin and joined to the heart by wires that measure the pulse and correct a heart rhythm that is too fast or too slow.

PACKED RED BLOOD CELLS (PRBCS) The blood product containing mostly red blood cells that is given as a transfusion; the plasma and other cells are removed.

PALLIATIVE CARE Care that treats a disease or its symptoms, providing relief but not necessarily a cure. The term is often used to describe end-of-life care. Palliation is sometimes called symptomatic treatment and relief. *See also* hospice.

PALPITATIONS A rapid, strong heartbeat. This is normal with fear, emotion, or exertion. It may also be a symptom of neurosis, arrhythmia, heart disease, or an overactive circulation (as in thyrotoxicosis).

PARALYSIS Loss of voluntary movement (motor function).

PAROXYSMAL ATRIAL TACHYCARDIA (PAT) The upper chambers of the heart beat abnormally fast.

PAT Paroxysmal atrial tachycardia; preadmission testing.

PATENT Open; unobstructed; affording free passage.

PATENT DUCTUS ARTERIOSUS (PDA) A congenital heart disease.

PATHOGEN An agent of disease, including bacteria, viruses, fungi, and protozoa.

PC After meals.

PDA Patent ductus arteriosis.

PE Physical examination.

PEAK-FLOW METER A hand-held device that measures airflow (how fast air is blown out of the lungs). Patients can use peak-flow meters to measure their own airflow, which allows asthmatic patients to predict an oncoming attack. *Peak flow* refers to the maximum flow rate of air breathed out during forced expiration.

PED Pediatric.

PEDIATRIC Pertaining to children.

PEG Percutaneous endoscopic gastrostomy.

PER OS By mouth.

PERCUTANEOUS ENDOSCOPIC GASTROSTOMY (PEG) A surgical procedure for placing a feeding tube without doing an open laparotomy (larger operation on the abdomen).

PERFUSION 1. The passage of fluid through a tissue, especially the passage of blood through the lung tissue to pick up oxygen from the air in the alveoli, which is brought there by ventilation. If ventilation is impaired, deoxygenated venous blood is returned to the general circulation, and insufficient gas exchange (oxygen for waste carbon dioxide) occurs. 2. The deliberate introduction of fluid into a tissue, usually by injection into the blood vessels supplying the tissue.

PERICARDIAL EFFUSION A condition in which fluid collects in the pericardial sac (the outer covering of the heart). The fluid, which may place pressure on the heart and cause it to pump ineffectively, can be drawn off by using a needle or by administering diuretics.

PERICARDITIS Inflammation of the pericardium, the fibrous membrane that surrounds the heart and its major blood vessels.

PERIODIC BREATHING Clusters of breaths separated by intervals of apnea (no breathing) or near apnea. Can be common in the elderly.

PERIPHERAL Away from the core. A *peripheral vascular disease* is a disease of the blood vessels in the extremities (arms and legs).

PERIPHERAL LINE An intravenous line placed in veins that are close to the skin surface. Used to deliver fluid or medications.

PERISTALSIS The rippling motion of muscles in the digestive tract, moving food through and, in the stomach, mixing food with gastric juices, turning it into a thin liquid.

PERITONEAL ADHESIONS The binding of abdominal organs to the peritoneum, a two-layered membrane that lines the wall of the abdominal cavity and covers the abdominal organs, a condition that can be repaired by surgery.

PERITONEAL DIALYSIS *See* dialysis.

PERITONITIS Inflammation of the peritoneum (the layer of cells lining the inner wall of the abdomen and pelvis). Peritonitis can result from infection, injury and bleeding, or disease.

PERL Pupils equal and reactive to light.

PERRLA Pupils equal, round, and reactive to light and accommodation (accommodation is how the eye accommodates and maintains focus on something like a moving finger). A test used in cases of suspected concussion.

PET SCAN Positron emission tomography.

PFT Pulmonary function test.

PH Measurement of acidity or alkalinity (concentration of hydrogen ions) on a seven-degree scale.

PHENOMENAL Occurring suddenly, unexpectedly, and even inexplicably. Example: "The patient started to bleed phenomenally."

PHYSICAL THERAPY (PT; IN CANADA: PHYSIOTHERAPY) Therapy to restore movement to limbs and muscles compromised by illness or injury.

PICC Percutaneously inserted central catheter. *See* central line.

PICU Pediatric intensive-care unit.

PIMU Pediatric intermediate-care or "step down" unit.

PLACEBO A medicine that is ineffective but that may help to relieve a condition because the patient has faith in its powers. New drugs are tested against placebos in clinical trials. The effect of a drug is compared with the placebo response, which occurs even in the absence of any pharmacologically active substance in the placebo.

PLASMA The liquid part of blood and lymphatic fluid. Plasma, which makes up about half of the volume of blood, contains antibodies and other proteins and does not clot. It is taken from donors and made into medications for a variety of blood-related conditions.

PLATELET A type of blood cell that is necessary to stop bleeding and allow injured areas to form clots. A normal adult platelet count is 150,000 – 400,000 platelets per microliter.

PLATELET COUNT A calculation of the number of platelets in a given volume of blood. Both increases and decreases can point to abnormal conditions, such as excess bleeding or clotting problems.

PMS Premenstrual syndrome.

PNEUMOMEDIASTINUM A collection of air in the central chest cavity.

PNEUMONECTOMY Surgical removal of all or part of a lung.

PNEUMONIA An inflammation of one or both lungs, frequently but not always due to infection. The infection may be bacterial, viral, fungal, or parasitic. Symptoms may include fever, chills, coughs with sputum production, chest pain, and shortness of breath.

PNEUMOTHORAX A condition in which free air is in the chest outside the lungs. It can occur spontaneously (with or without an underlying lung disease) or following a fractured rib or following chest surgery, or it can be deliberately induced in order to collapse the lung. A small pneumothorax without an underlying lung disease may resolve on its own. A larger pneumothorax or one associated with an underlying lung disease often requires aspiration of the free air and/or placement of a chest tube to evacuate the air and allow lungs to reexpand.

PO By mouth (Latin: *per os*).

POSITRON EMISSION TOMOGRAPHY (PET) A new scanning technology that assesses internal tissues and organs and produces three-dimensional color-coded images that assist in diagnosis.

POST-ANESTHESIA CARE UNIT The area to which a patient is brought to recover from surgery. Also called the recovery room.

POST-OP Postoperative.

PREMATURE ATRIAL CONTRACTION (PAC) Heart contractions that occur too early in the rhythm sequence.

PREMATURE VENTRICULAR CONTRACTION (PVC) Premature heartbeats originating from the ventricles and occurring before the regular heartbeat.

PREMENSTRUAL SYNDROME (PMS) A collection of physical and emotional discomforts (including cramps, irritability, and bloating) typically occurring one to two weeks prior to a woman's period.

PRE-OP Preoperative.

PREP Prepare.

PRESCRIPTION A doctor's order for the preparation and administration of a drug or device for a patient.

PRESENT To manifest. Used by health-care providers in formal reports, as in "The patient presented with confusion and severe abdominal bruising."

PRESSOR Agent used to cause a rise in blood pressure.

PRIMARY 1. Referring to a doctor who is principally responsible for the overall care of a patient. 2. Referring to the original source of a cancer that may have spread to another part of the body.

PRN As needed; when necessary; when requested (Latin: *pro re nata*).

PROCEDURE A series of actions to be executed in the same manner, with the goal of achieving the same result in the same circumstances every time—for example, hospital emergency procedures and routine bedside tasks.

PROGNOSIS The probable outcome or course of a disease and the chance of recovery.

PROGRESSIVE Increasing in scope or severity. A disease that is progressive is going from bad to worse.

PROM Passive range of motion.

PRONE Lying on the stomach.

PRONOUNCE To officially state (the time of death). When a person dies in the hospital, a doctor must formally pronounce the person dead and then state (or "call") the time of death for the hospital records, as well as for legal purposes.

PROPHYLACTIC A preventive measure taken in an attempt to fend off a disease or another unwanted consequence.

PROSTATECTOMY Surgery for the partial or complete removal of the prostate.

PROSTHESIS An artificial substitute or replacement of a part of the body, such as a tooth, eye, hip, knee, leg, or arm. A prosthesis is designed for functional and/or cosmetic reasons.

PROTOCOL A defined way of doing things. In the hospital, a protocol is based on evidence (past clinical research) or medical guidelines and set down in a printed set of instructions on how particular medical situations are to be dealt with.

PRURITUS Itching caused by a drug reaction, food allergy, kidney or liver disease, cancer, parasite, aging or dry skin, a contact skin reaction (to poison ivy, for example), or an unknown agent.

PT Patient.

PT Physical therapy; (in Canada:) physiotherapy.

PTA Prior to admission (to the hospital).

PULMONARY Having to do with the lungs.

PULSE The rhythmic dilation of an artery in response to the beating of the heart. Pulse is often measured by feeling the wrist, then by counting the number of dilations that occur within ten seconds and multiplying that number by six. The result is the heart rate (number of beats per minute).

PULSE OXIMETER A sensor placed on the hand or foot of a patient to monitor the concentration of oxygen in the blood.

PUS A thick whitish yellow fluid that results from the accumulation of white blood cells, liquefied tissue, and cellular debris. Pus is common at a site of infection or foreign material in the body.

PVC Premature ventricular contraction.

PWB Partial weight bearing (said of a leg).

PYLORIC STENOSIS Narrowing (stenosis) of the outlet of the stomach so that food cannot pass easily from the stomach into the duodenum (intestine), resulting in feeding problems and projectile vomiting. The obstruction can be corrected by a simple surgical procedure.

Q Each, every (Latin: *quaque*).

QD Every day (Latin: *quaque die*).

QH Every hour (Latin: *quaque hora*). Thus, *q2h, q3h,* etc., mean "every two hours," "every three hours," etc.

QID Four times daily (Latin: *quater in die*).

QNS Quantity not sufficient.

QOD Every other day (Latin: *quater otra die*).

QS Sufficient quantity (Latin: *quantum sufficiat*).

QT Quart.

QUADRANT Quarter. For example, the liver is in the right upper quadrant of the abdomen.

QUADRIPLEGIA Paralysis of all four limbs, resulting from a spinal cord accident or a stroke.

QUALITY OF LIFE The ability to enjoy normal life activities—an important consideration in medical care. Some medical treatments can seriously impair quality of life without providing benefits, whereas others greatly enhance quality of life.

RADIATION THERAPY (RT) Treatment using high-energy radiation. The use of high-energy rays damages cancer cells, stopping them from growing and dividing. Like surgery, radiation therapy is a local treatment that affects cancer cells only in the treated area. Radiation can come from a machine (external radiation) or from a small container of radioactive material implanted directly into or near the tumor (internal radiation).

RANGE OF MOTION (ROM) 1. The range through which a joint can be moved, both flexed and extended, as measured in degrees—for example, a knee may lack 10 degrees of full extension. 2. The movement of joints through their range of motion by a therapist or nurse to preserve their function for patients having prolonged bed rest.

RASH A breakout on the skin; exanthem.

RBCS Red blood cells.

RECIPIENT Someone who receives something, such as a blood transfusion or an organ transplant.

RECURRENCE The return of a sign, symptom, or disease after a remission. The reappearance of cancer cells at the same site or in another location is a familiar form of recurrence.

RED BLOOD (ARTERIAL BLOOD) Blood pumped by the heart through the lungs, where it will pick up oxygen and circulate through the body in the arteries. *See also* blue blood.

RED BLOOD CELL (RBC) COUNT A calculation of the number of red blood cells per volume of blood. Both increases and decreases can point to abnormal conditions.

RED BLOOD CELLS (RBCS) Cells in the blood that carry oxygen to tissues in the body.

REFERRAL The recommendation to make an appointment with a medical or paramedical professional.

REFLEX A reaction that is involuntary. The corneal reflex is the blink that occurs when the eye is irritated. The nasal reflex is a sneeze.

REFLUX The backing up of a liquid—for example, into the esophagus from the stomach or into ducts from the bladder.

REFRACTORY Not yielding or improving with treatment or therapy— for example, otitis that is refractory to penicillin.

REGIMEN A regulated diet, exercise, treatment, or other course designed to give a good result. A low-salt diet is a regimen.

REGIONAL ANESTHETIC An anesthetic used to numb a portion of the body.

REGISTERED NURSE (RN) A nurse who has graduated from an accredited nursing program, has passed the state or provincial license exam, and is registered and licensed to practice by a state or provincial authority.

REGRESS 1. To return or go back, particularly to return to a pattern of behavior or level of skill characteristic of a person at a younger age. Regression sometimes occurs in the elderly. 2. To worsen (in reference to a disease).

REGURGITATION A backward flow—for example, a regurgitation of food (causing vomiting) or a regurgitation of blood (the sloshing of blood back into the heart or between chambers of the heart when a heart valve is faulty and does not close effectively).

REHAB Rehabilitation.

REHABILITATION (REHAB) The restoration of skills to a person who has had an illness or injury by using physical therapy and occupational therapy, among other techniques. The goal is to help the patient regain maximum self-sufficiency and the ability to function in as normal (or as near normal) a manner as possible.

REJECTION The refusal by the body to accept transplanted cells, tissues, or organs. For example, a kidney transplant may be rejected.

RELAPSE The return of a disease and its signs and symptoms after the patient has enjoyed a remission. Also known as a recurrence.

REMIFENTANIL A pain reliever for inducing and maintaining general anesthesia during surgery. The drug breaks down in the bloodstream and body tissues very quickly and safely. Because enzymes break down remifentanil in the blood and muscles, rather than in the liver and kidneys, like other drugs, patients wake sooner, and breathing tubes can be removed sooner.

REMISSION Disappearance of the signs and symptoms of cancer or another disease. When this happens, the disease is said to be "in remission." A remission can be temporary or permanent. *See also* spontaneous remission.

RENAL Having to do with the kidneys. In a case of renal failure the kidneys have stopped functioning.

RESECTION Surgical removal of part of an organ. *See also* wedge resection of the lung.

RESIDENTS Doctors in a hospital completing specialized training. They participate in a patient's care under the direction of a primary doctor.

RESIDUAL Left behind or remaining after recovery from an illness or injury—for example, a residual ache.

RESISTANCE Opposition to something or the ability to withstand it. For example, some forms of bacterial infection are resistant to treatment with penicillin.

RESP Respiration.

RESPIRATION ("RESP") The act of inhaling and exhaling air in order to exchange oxygen for carbon dioxide.

RESPIRATOR *See* ventilator.

RESPIRATORY SYNCYTIAL VIRUS (RSV) A virus that causes mild respiratory infections (colds and coughs) in adults but that can produce severe respiratory problems (bronchiolitis and pneumonia) in young children.

RESPIRATORY THERAPIST (RT) A specially trained therapist who helps to promote, improve, or maintain the health of the lungs by administering breathing treatments and managing ventilators, among other functions.

RESPONSE A patient's reaction or lack of reaction to drugs or therapy. Example: "She is not responding well to antibiotics."

RETENTION Holding in. *Urine retention* is the lack of ability to urinate.

RISK FACTOR Something (smoking; excessive alcohol consumption) that increases a person's chances of developing a disease.

RISK OF RECURRENCE 1. In medical genetics: the chance that a genetic (inherited) disease present in a family will recur in the family. 2. In general medicine: the chance that an illness may recur in an individual.

RN Registered nurse.

R/O Rule out.

ROM Range of motion.

ROUNDS In most hospitals, daily visits to each patient by the patient's primary doctor to review the cases and assess progress. If the hospital is a teaching facility, the doctor may be accompanied by medical students, interns, or residents, as well as by other members of the clinical team.

R/R Respiratory rate.

RR Recovery room.

RT Radiation therapy.

RT Right.

RTC Return to clinic.

RX Prescription, treatment, or therapy.

S Without (Latin: *sine*).

SALINE Relating to salt. In medicine, a saline solution is a salt solution that is adjusted to the normal salinity of the human body. Certain concentrations of both sodium and chloride in the blood are essential for normal body functions. Solutions containing sodium chloride (salt) and sterile water are commonly used as fluid replacements to treat or prevent dehydration and are often administered intravenously.

SALPINGECTOMY Surgical removal of a fallopian tube.

SCOPOLAMINE PATCH A prescription drug that helps prevent nausea and vomiting associated with motion sickness. The patch is now being used to prevent nausea and vomiting during or after surgery—which is important to prevent aspiration (the inhalation of gastric contents into the lungs and the lower airways). The small patch is placed behind the ear the night before surgery, allowing medication to be absorbed through the skin and travel directly into the bloodstream.

SCRUBS Standard clothing—gowns, or shirts and trousers—worn by surgeons and surgical staff. The name probably originates from the need to scrub hands and forearms before surgery. Also called greens in some hospitals, a name originating from their usually green color, chosen because it contrasts with the sterile white environment of the operating room, reduces eye fatigue, and makes red blood splashes less conspicuous than they appear on the traditional plain white scrubs.

SEDATIVE A drug that calms a patient, easing agitation and permitting sleep. Often used prior to procedures such as MRIs and CT scans.

SEIZURE DISORDER A medical condition characterized by episodes of uncontrolled electrical activity in the brain (seizures). Most seizures last from thirty seconds to two minutes and do not cause lasting harm. Frequent seizures with unconsciousness between them and seizures that last longer than five minutes are considered medical emergencies. A pattern of seizures is often referred to as epilepsy. Possible causes include hereditary or genetic factors, birth defects, head injuries, brain tumors, and infectious diseases like encephalitis and meningitis.

SENSORY 1. Relating to sensation—that is, the perception of a stimulus and the reaction of nerve impulses in the nerve centers. 2. Relating to the senses themselves.

SEPSIS, SEPTICEMIA The spread of bacteria or other microorganisms and their toxins from a site of infection to the bloodstream; a bloodstream infection. Sepsis may be associated with clinical symptoms of systemic (bodywide) illness, such as fever, chills, malaise, low blood pressure, and changes in mental status. It can be a life-threatening disease, calling for urgent and comprehensive care. Treatment depends on the type of infection but usually begins with antibiotics or similar medications. Sepsis is also known as blood poisoning.

SEPTIC Relating to sepsis, a widespread, systemic illness caused by a local infection that spreads to the blood and that can eventually involve the entire body.

SEPTICEMIA See sepsis.

SEPTOSTOMY Surgical incision of a hole in the septum, the wall between the left and right chambers of the heart, usually done to increase blood flow through the lungs.

SERUM The clear liquid that can be separated from clotted blood. The clot makes the difference between serum and plasma, which is the liquid portion of normal unclotted blood that contains the red and white blood cells and platelets.

SERVICE A division of the hospital medical staff devoted to a particular specialty.

SHARPS Needles, scalpels, and other sharp instruments that are considered dangerous and that must be handled with extreme caution.

SHEARING A tearing or stretching of nerves or brain tissue that results when the brain twists and hits against the skull. Shearing is usually caused by a sudden deceleration or a stop, like that involved in a car accident.

SHOCK A critical condition brought on by a sudden drop in blood flow, oxygen, or glucose in the body. When the circulatory system fails to maintain adequate blood flow and oxygenation, this sharply cuts back the delivery of oxygen and nutrients to vital organs, compromising the kidneys and curtailing the removal of wastes from the body. *Hypovolemic shock* is caused by a drop in blood volume. *Cardiogenic shock* is caused by a drop in output of blood by the heart. The signs and symptoms of shock include low blood pressure (hypotension), hyperventilation, a weak, rapid pulse, cold, clammy grayish bluish (cyanotic) skin, decreased urine flow (oliguria), and mental changes (anxiety and foreboding, confusion, and sometimes combativeness). Shock is a major medical emergency. It is common after serious injury. Emergency care for shock includes giving fluids or blood intravenously, medications to help the heart, and often oxygen.

SHUNT A tube or pathway that diverts blood or another body fluid through an alternate route inside the body.

SIDE EFFECT An unwanted effect produced by a drug in addition to its desired therapeutic effect. Drug manufacturers are required to list all known side effects of their products. When the side effects of a necessary medication are potentially severe, sometimes a second medication, lifestyle change, dietary change, or other measure may help to minimize them.

SIGMOIDOSCOPY A test that uses a thin flexible tube with a light at the end (a sigmoidoscope) to inspect the rectum and lower large intestine for abnormalities.

SKULL FRACTURE A break in one or more of the bones of the skull.

SLEEP APNEA A disorder characterized by interruptions of breathing during sleep. *Central sleep apnea* occurs when the brain fails to send the right signals to the breathing muscles to start breathing. *Obstructive sleep apnea* occurs when air cannot flow into or out of the person's nose or mouth, although efforts to breathe continue. Obstructive sleep apnea is much more common than central sleep apnea. In obstructive sleep apnea, the throat collapses or is obstructed during sleep, causing the individual to snort and gasp for breath. Hundreds of these episodes can occur every night, causing daytime sleepiness and even increasing the risk of hypertension and heart problems. An *apnea monitor,* which monitors breathing patterns through electrode patches placed on the chest, sounds an alarm if the time between breaths becomes too long.

SM Small.

SNF Skilled-nursing facility.

SOB Shortness of breath.

SOMATIC NERVOUS SYSTEM The part of the nervous system that uses external stimuli (sight, hearing, touch) to control voluntary movements through the action of skeletal muscles. *See also* autonomic nervous system.

SOMNOLENT Sleepy or tending to cause sleepiness.

S/P Status post. Used to alert others on the health-care team to recent surgeries (or conditions) a patient may have had.

SPASM A brief automatic jerking movement. A muscle spasm can be quite painful, with the muscle clenching tightly. Spasms may be caused by stress, medication, overexercise, or other factors.

SPASTICITY A state of increased tone of a muscle (and an increase in the deep tendon reflexes). With spasticity of the legs (spastic paraplegia) the leg muscles feel tight and rigid, and the knee jerk reflex is exaggerated.

SPINAL ANESTHETIC An anesthetic that is injected into the spinal canal fluid before surgery in the lower abdomen, pelvis, rectum, or other lower extremities.

SPLENECTOMY Surgical removal of the spleen.

SPONTANEOUS REMISSION Any recovery from illness that appears to have occurred without medical treatment.

SPRAIN An injury to a ligament resulting from overuse or trauma. The treatment of a sprain injury includes ice packs, rest and elevation of the involved joint, anti-inflammatory medications, support bracing, and only gradual return to activity affecting the ligament. Local cortisone injections are sometimes given for persistent inflammation. The application of ice after activity can reduce or prevent recurrent inflammation. In severe sprains, an orthopedic surgical repair may be performed.

SPUTUM The mucus material from the lungs that a person coughs up.

STAPH Staphylococcal, staphylococcus.

STAPHYLOCOCCUS (**"STAPH"**) A bacterium normally found on the skin and in the mucus that may cause infection.

STAT Immediately; right away (Latin: *statim*).

STD Sexually transmitted disease.

STEM CELLS The youngest bone marrow cells, from which other marrow cells are formed.

STENOSIS A narrowing. *Aortic stenosis* is a narrowing of the aortic valve in the heart. *Pulmonary stenosis* is a narrowing of the pulmonary valve in the heart. *Pyloric stenosis* is a narrowing of the outlet of the stomach.

STENT A tube designed to be inserted into a blood vessel or passageway to keep it open, acting like miniature scaffolding. Often used in cases of advanced heart disease.

STEROID A large group of substances with the same chemical framework and a related structure. Many hormones, body cells, and drugs are steroids—for example, prednisone (a drug used to relieve swelling and inflammation) and testosterone (the principal male hormone).

STETHOSCOPE An instrument used to transmit low-volume sounds such as the heartbeat and intestinal and lung sounds to the ear of the listener.

STOMA A hole; commonly, the hole that allows feces out from the colon and into a colostomy bag.

STREP *Streptococcus.*

STREPTOCOCCUS (**"STREP"**) A type of bacteria that causes infection—for example, strep throat.

STROKE A rapid loss of brain function due to an interruption of blood supply to the brain. A stroke can cause permanent neurological damage and even death.

SUBCUTANEOUS Under the skin. With a subcutaneous injection, the needle of a syringe is inserted just under the skin to deliver a medication, as opposed to delivery into the skin (intradermal), into a muscle (intramuscular), or into a vein (intravenous).

SUCTION Removal of mucus and fluid from the nose, mouth, or endotracheal tube.

SUPERIOR VENA CAVA (SVC) The large vein responsible for bringing blood back to the heart after it has circulated to the brain and upper body.

SUPINE Lying on the back, face up.

SUPPORTIVE CARE Treatment given to prevent, control, or relieve complications and side effects and to improve the patient's comfort and quality of life.

SVC Superior vena cava.

SWAB A pad of absorbent material (such as cotton), sometimes attached to a stick or wire, used for cleaning out or applying medication to wounds, operation sites, or body cavities. Also used for lab tests.

SX Symptoms.

SYMPATHETIC NERVOUS SYSTEM The part of the nervous system over which a person does not have conscious control. This includes nerves of the heart and lungs.

SYMPTOM Any abnormal change in appearance, sensation, or function that indicates a disease process.

SYNCOPE Loss of consciousness ("passing out") induced by a temporarily insufficient flow of blood to the brain. Syncope, which is not uncommon in otherwise healthy people, may be caused by an emotional shock, by standing for prolonged periods, by injury, and by profuse bleeding.

SYNDROME A combination of signs and symptoms that occur together and characterize a particular disease, illness, or abnormality.

SYRINGE A device used to inject fluid into or withdraw fluid from the body. In a syringe a needle is attached to a hollow cylinder that is fitted with a sliding plunger. The downward movement of the plunger injects fluid; upward movement withdraws fluid.

SYSTEMIC THERAPY Treatment that reaches cells throughout the body by traveling through the bloodstream.

SYSTOLIC BLOOD PRESSURE The blood pressure rate when the heart is contracting, specifically the maximum arterial pressure during contraction of the left ventricle of the heart. The time when a ventricular contraction occurs is called systole. In a blood pressure reading, the systolic pressure is typically the first number recorded. With a blood pressure of 120/80, the systolic pressure is 120.

T Temperature.

T & A Tonsillectomy and adenoidectomy.

TAB Tablet.

TACHYCARDIA Fast, above-normal heartbeat.

TACHYPNEA Abnormally fast breathing.

TACTILE Having to do with touch.

TB Tuberculosis.

TBSP Tablespoon.

THERAPEUTIC Relating to the beneficial treatment of disease; healthy. The therapeutic dose of a drug is the amount needed to treat a disease. A diet high in fiber is therapeutic.

THERAPY The treatment of a disease or a condition.

THORACOTOMY Surgery to view the lung, used to confirm the presence of cancer or, in case of chest trauma, to detect the source of bleeding.

THROMBOLYTIC DRUG Medication used to dissolve blood clots.

THROMBOSIS The formation or presence of a clot within a blood vessel, which can block the flow of blood through the circulatory system.

TIA Transient ischemia attack. *See* ischemia.

TID Three times a day (Latin: *ter in die*). Sometimes "three times a day" is written as q8h, "every eight hours."

TISSUE A broad term applied to any group of cells that perform specific functions—for example, the skin.

TLC Total lung capacity.

TONSILLECTOMY AND ADENOIDECTOMY (T & A) Surgical removal of the tonsils and adenoids.

TOPICAL Applied to a certain area of the skin and intended to affect only the area to which it is applied. An ointment can be topical.

TOTAL HYSTERECTOMY *See* hysterectomy.

TOTAL PARENTERAL NUTRITION (TPN) A technique for meeting a patient's nutritional needs by means of intravenous feedings. TPN provides proteins, fats, carbohydrates, water, electrolytes, vitamins, and minerals needed for the building of tissue, expenditure of energy, and healing. It is sometimes called hyperalimentation, even though it does not provide excessive ("hyper") amounts of nutrients.

TPN Total parenteral nutrition.

TPR Temperature, pulse, respiration.

TRACHEA Windpipe.

TRACHEOSTOMY, TRACHEOTOMY ("TRACH") A surgical hole is cut into the windpipe for a tube to assist with breathing. The tube, which is frequently attached to a ventilator, is usually inserted if a patient will need a ventilator for a long time, has an injury to the face or neck that makes breathing difficult, or has an obstruction of the upper airway. Health-care providers may refer to "a trach," or to a patient as "trached."

TRACTION, ORTHOPEDIC The use of a system of weights and pulleys to change the position of a bone over time. Traction may be used in cases of bone injury or congenital defect to prevent scar tissue from building up in ways to limit movement and to prevent contractures (permanent shortening of tissues such as muscles) in disorders such as cerebral palsy and arthritis.

TRAIT Any genetically determined characteristic, such as eye color and hair color.

TRANSFUSION The transfer of blood or blood products from one person (the donor) into the bloodstream of another person (the recipient). In most situations, this is done as a lifesaving maneuver to replace blood cells or blood products lost through severe bleeding. Transfusion of the patient's own blood (autologous or auto transfusion) is the safest method to replace the blood, but that requires planning ahead, and not all patients are eligible. Directed donor blood allows the patient to receive blood from known donors.

TRANSIENT ISCHEMIC ATTACK (TIA) Informally called a "mini stroke." a TIA lasts only a few minutes but with effects (confusion, numbness, dizziness, difficulty speaking) that may persist up to twenty-four hours.

TRANSILLUMINATION The passing of a strong beam of light through a part of the body for clinical inspection.

TRANSPLANT The grafting of tissue or an organ from one place to another. The transplant can be from one part of the body to another (autologous transplantation), as in the case of a skin graft using the patient's own skin, or from one patient to another (allogenic transplantation), as in the case of transplanting a donor kidney into a recipient.

TRAUMA Any injury, whether physically or emotionally inflicted. Medically, trauma refers to a serious or critical bodily injury, wound, illness, or shock. Severity and prognoses are measured according to a numerical scale (a trauma score). Psychologically, trauma refers to an experience that is emotionally painful, distressful, or shocking, which often results in lasting mental and physical effects.

TREMOR An abnormal repetitive shaking movement of the body or a part of the body. Tremors can be genetic or related to illnesses (such as thyroid disease), fever, drugs, or being cold or afraid.

TRIAGE The process of sorting patients based on their need for immediate medical treatment as compared to their chance of benefiting from such care. Triage is done in emergency rooms, during major disasters, and in wars when limited medical resources must be allocated to maximize the number of survivors.

TSP Teaspoon.

TUBE FEED The patient's food and medications are delivered via a tube inserted through the nose or mouth directly into the stomach or small intestine.

TUBERCULOSIS (TB) An infectious inflammatory disease that must be reported to public health authorities. It is chronic in nature and commonly affects the lungs (pulmonary tuberculosis), although it may occur in almost any part of the body. The causative agent is *Mycobacterium tuberculosis.*

TUMOR An abnormal mass of tissue. Tumors, a classic sign of inflammation, can be benign or malignant (cancerous). There are dozens of different types of tumors. Their names usually reflect the kind of tissue they arise in, and may also tell something about their shape or how they grow.

TX Treatment.

TYMPANIC MEMBRANE Eardrum.

UA Urinalysis.

UGI Upper gastrointestinal.

ULCER Tissue erosion of an area of the skin or the lining of the gastrointestinal (GI) tract. An ulcer is always depressed below the level of the surrounding tissue. Ulcers on the skin are often due to irritation, as with bedsores, and they may become infected and inflamed as they grow.

ULTRASOUND High-frequency sound waves. Ultrasound waves can be bounced off tissues using special devices, and the echoes can be converted into pictures called sonograms. *Ultrasound imaging,* or ultrasonography, allows doctors and patients to get an inside view of soft tissues and body cavities without using invasive techniques. Ultrasound is often used to examine a fetus during pregnancy.

UNCONSCIOUSNESS Interruption of a person's awareness of self and surroundings; inability to notice or respond to stimuli in the environment. A person may become unconscious because of oxygen deprivation, shock, central nervous system depressants (such as alcohol and drugs), or injury. In psychology, the unconscious is that part of thought and emotion that happens outside everyday awareness but may affect it.

UPPER GASTROINTESTINAL SERIES (UPPER GI SERIES) A series of tests of the upper and middle portions of the gastrointestinal tract. The person being tested swallows a "shake" of barium and water (barium contrast material), then gas-producing crystals. The doctor tracks the progress of the barium through the esophagus, stomach, and small intestine using a fluoroscope connected to a video monitor. Several X-ray pictures are usually taken at different times and from different directions.

UPPER RESPIRATORY INFECTION (URI) An infection often caused by a virus of the upper part of the breathing system, including the nose, throat, and upper portion of the bronchi (bronchial tubes—the breathing tubes of the lungs).

URETERS Ducts that carry urine from the kidneys to the bladder.

URI Upper respiratory infection.

URINALYSIS (UA) A test that determines the content of the urine. Because urine removes toxins and excess liquids from the body, urinalysis can be used to detect some types of disease, particularly in the case of bladder or kidney infections, metabolic disorders, and kidney disease, and to uncover evidence of drug use.

URINARY RETENTION Inability to empty the bladder.

URINARY TRACT The entire system of ducts and channels that conduct urine from the kidneys to the exterior of the body. It includes the ureters, the bladder, and the urethra (the canal from the bladder to outside).

URINARY TRACT INFECTION (UTI) A bacterial infection of the urinary tract, most often caused by the bacterium *Escherichia coli* (*E. coli*). Urinary tract infections are more common in women than in men. They usually affect the bladder (cystitis), but can also affect the kidneys (pyelonephritis). The symptoms at first are usually frequent urination, an urgent need to urinate, and pain with urination (dysuria). The symptoms may also include fever, cloudy urine, foul-smelling urine, or blood in the urine (hematuria). If the infection affects the kidneys, the symptoms will usually also include high fever, chills, back pain on the side of the affected kidney, nausea, and vomiting.

UROSTOMY An opening created in the body to provide a new path for the evacuation of urine.

URTICARIA Hives—raised, itchy areas of skin that are usually a sign of an allergic reaction. Hives typically last less than four hours, but they may stay for days or weeks. Approximately 20 percent of people have experienced a bout of urticaria.

UTERUS A hollow, muscular organ of the female reproductive system.

UTI Urinary tract infection.

VACCINATION Injection of a killed or incapacitated microbe or toxin in order to stimulate the immune system against the microbe or toxin, thereby preventing the occurrence of the disease that the active microbe or toxin can cause.

VAS CATH A temporary central venous catheter that is used for leukopheresis (removing white cells from the blood) or dialysis procedures. It is usually inserted into a large vein in the neck, chest, or groin.

VASODILATORS Drugs that relax the smooth muscles in blood vessels, causing the vessels to dilate and leading to an increase in blood flow.

VENOUS Referring to veins. *See also* blue blood.

VENTILATOR A machine (often called a respirator) that is designed to assist or take over breathing for a patient. The ventilator has many different settings or capabilities (modes) to provide optimal breathing assistance. Ventilators come equipped with noisy alarms to alert the medical staff to potential problems.

VENTRICLE A chamber, or hollow space, of an organ. The four connected cavities in the central portion of the brain and the lower two chambers of the heart are called ventricles.

VENTRICULAR FIBRILLATION ("VEE-FIB") A state in which the heart's muscles move chaotically and without purpose, thus preventing delivery of blood to the body. If not reversed, ventricular fibrillation can lead to death.

VENTRICULAR SEPTAL DEFECT (VSD) A congenital defect in the septum of the heart.

VERTEBRA A vertebra is one of thirty-three bony segments that form the spinal column of a human being. There are seven cervical (neck), twelve thoracic (between neck and abdomen), five lumbar (between abdomen and sacrum), five sacral (fused into one sacrum bone in the pelvis), and four coccygeal (fused into one coccyx, or tailbone) vertebrae.

VERTIGO Dizziness; a disabling sensation in which affected individuals feel that either they or their surroundings are in constant movement—most often a spinning motion, but the ground may also seem to be tilting. Vertigo is usually due to a problem with the inner ear but can also be caused by brain stem problems.

VIRUS A microorganism that cannot grow or reproduce apart from a living cell but that causes many human infections and diseases. A virus invades cells and uses their chemical machinery to keep itself alive and to replicate itself. It may reproduce with fidelity (its "offspring" are identically the same) or with errors (mutations), which can be difficult to identify and then treat.

VITAL SIGNS (VS) Signs of life; the most basic body functions—temperature, pulse, respiratory rate, and blood pressure—which can be measured either manually or by machine.

VITAL SIGNS ABSENT (VSA) Clinically dead. The term is used to denote the absence of a heartbeat or breathing.

VOL Volume.

VS Vital signs.

VSA Vital signs absent.

VSD Ventricular septal defect.

W/ With.

WB Weight bearing.

WBCS White blood cells.

W/C Wheelchair.

WEDGE RESECTION OF THE LUNG Removal of a small section of the lung, often for a lung biopsy.

WHEEZING A whistling noise in the chest during breathing when the airways are narrowed or compressed, as in asthma or bronchiolitis.

WHITE BLOOD CELL (WBC) COUNT A calculation of the number of white blood cells per volume of blood. Both increases and decreases can be significant.

WHITE BLOOD CELLS (WBCS) Cells found in the blood and in tissues that aid in fighting infections and making antibodies for the immune system's attack on disease. There are several types of white blood cells, including neutrophils and lymphocytes.

WITHDRAWAL SYMPTOMS Abnormal physical or psychological reactions that follow the abrupt stoppage of a drug that has produced physical dependence (addiction). Common withdrawal symptoms include sweating, tremors, vomiting, anxiety, insomnia, fever, irritability, and muscle pain.

WNL Within normal limits.

W/O Without.

WT Weight.

X-MATCH Cross-matching (of blood).

XR X-ray.

X-RAY A form of radiation, like light or radio waves, that can be focused into a beam, much like a flashlight beam. X-rays can pass through most objects, including the human body. When X-rays strike a piece of photographic film, they can produce a picture that is useful in making medical diagnoses. Dense tissues in the body, such as bones, block (absorb) many of the X-rays and appear white on an X-ray picture. Less dense tissues, such as muscles and organs, block fewer of the X-rays (more of the X-rays pass through) and appear in shades of gray. X-rays that pass only through air appear black.

YEAST *Candida albicans* is a yeast—a fungal organism—that is present in the natural flora of the mouth, gastrointestinal tract, and skin. Normally the body's natural defenses keep it in check. When fungal growth exceeds the body's ability to control it, a yeast infection develops—called thrush (visible as white patches) when it is present in the mouth and throat. It is very common among hospital patients who have been on certain long-term antibiotics. A yeast infection can also develop when the immune system is weakened by illness or stress.

YO Year old.

YR Year.

ZINC A mineral essential to the body. Zinc is a constituent of many enzymes that permit chemical reactions to proceed at normal rates. It is involved in the manufacture of protein (protein synthesis) and cell division, and a serious zinc deficiency can result in the loss of a person's sense of smell. Zinc is also a constituent of insulin.

Staff Slang: What You Might Overhear

Some words, acronyms, euphemisms, and phrases that might be overheard in hospital wards aren't in the glossy hospital brochures. Administrators, boards, and public relations staff want to pretend they don't exist. But they do. They're used every day by doctors, nurses, paramedics, and other personnel directly involved in care, but their usage can vary from hospital to hospital—or even from country to country, depending on the local slang vocabulary.

At one time, these words routinely turned up in official medical records as off-the-wall treatment orders, pessimistic diagnoses, and disparaging comments about troublesome patients—the scribbled entries were in a kind of irreverent shorthand intended only for clinical insiders. That subversive practice ended abruptly with legislation that opened patients' medical records to the patients themselves. Some, horrified and insulted by what they read, launched formal complaints that quickly sent an entire lexicon scampering underground.

Such staff lingo, however unethical (never mind politically incorrect), still survives in whispered hallway exchanges, off-duty conversations, informal notes, and personal e-mails. If you spend time in the hospital and keep your eyes and ears open, you may gain some revealing insights about the people under those crisp uniforms and dispassionate veneers.

Some of the slang reflects the gallows humor that you might expect from people who have to deal constantly with injury, disease, and death. Some of it is downright offensive and demeaning. Some of it reflects anger and discouragement. Some of it seems wacky but has become useful shorthand, condensing personal opinions into brief exclamations. All of it is valuable to know because it collects into a portrait of people who seldom come out from behind their self-protective facades. Now you can know how they really feel and think. Note, for instance, the large number of euphemisms and acronyms for death. The professionals seem to have as much trouble dealing with unpleasant truths as the rest of us do.

WARNING: The following list contains words and phrases that some readers will find downright offensive. Discretion is advised.

3H ENEMA An enema that is High, Hot, and a Hell of a lot. Reputedly administered to patients who give staff a hard time.

3P'S Pill, Permissiveness, and Promiscuity. Used to describe a female patient with a sexually transmitted disease.

4F Fat, Fortyish, Flatulent, Female. Used to describe a stereotypical candidate for a diagnosis of gallbladder disease.

45C Said when the patient is one chromosome short of a full set; stupid.

5-H-1-T Polite term for shit.

(10TH) FLOOR TRANSFER A death. The floor number is the next number above the highest floor in the hospital.

ACUTE HYPONICOTAEMIA Nicotine addiction. Said of a patient desperate for a cigarette.

ACUTE LEAD POISONING Gunshot wound.

ADMINISPHERE Where hospital managers work, reckoned to be "another planet."

ADR Ain't Doing Right.

AFU & BR All Fucked Up and Beyond Repair.

AGA Acute Gravity Attack (fell over).

AGGRESSIVE EUTHANASIA Recommended as a procedure that obnoxious patients would benefit from.

AGMI Ain't Gonna Make It (won't survive).

AHF Acute Hissy Fit.

AIR BISCUIT A stool that floats.

ALBATROSS A chronically ill patient who will remain with a doctor until one or the other expires.

ALC A La Casa (send the patient home).

ALS Absolute Loss of Sanity (nutcase).

AMYOYO Adios, Motherfucker, You're On Your Own. 1. A comment about patients who sign out against medical advice. 2. A parting wisecrack from one doctor leaving a shift to another who has to remain. 3. A reaction to a very severe condition, such as a major head wound, for which the only medical option is to watch and wait.

ANGEL LUST 1. Used to describe a male cadaver with an erection (a state not uncommon after a traumatic death). 2. Used to describe death that occurred during sexual intercourse.

APD Acute Prozac Deficiency (depression).

APPY A person with suspected appendicitis.

APTFRAN Apply Pillow To Face, Repeat As Necessary. Said of an annoying patient.

AQP Assuming the Q Position (deteriorating or dying with the tongue hanging out).

AQR Ain't Quite Right.

ART Assuming Room Temperature (dead).

ASSMOSIS Promotion by kissing ass.

AST Assuming Seasonal Temperature (dead).

ATD Acute Tylenol Deficiency (simple fever or head cold).

ATFO Asked To Fuck Off.

AUNT MINNIE LESION Used in radiology to characterize a lesion that has a very unusual (even startling) appearance.

AXE A surgeon.

B & T *See* bagged and tagged.

BABY CATCHER An obstetrician.

BABY DOLL Vaginal bleeder.

BABYGRAM X-ray of a newborn.

BAG 'EM To put someone on a ventilator (respirator).

BAGGED AND TAGGED (B & T) A body in a bag and with a toe tag, ready for dispatch to the morgue.

BANANA A patient with jaundice.

BANANA BAGS IV bags containing a yellow fluid with vitamins, thiamine, and dextrose, given to chronic alcoholics whose electrolytes are depleted.

BAT Blunt Abdominal Trauma.

BBCS Bumps, Bruises, Cuts, and Scrapes. Indicates that there are no serious injuries.

BBL SIGN Belly Button Lint sign. Refers to a male who is middle-aged, overweight, and hairy. A belly button that looks like the lint trap in a clothes dryer is most common in overweight, hairy, older men.

BEACHED WHALE An obese patient unable to do much for himself or herself except lie there with flailing arms and legs.

BEAN Kidney.

BFH Big Fucking Head. 1. Water on the brain. Sometimes used in the expression "FLK with BFH." 2. An arrogant specialist. 3. Brat From Hell. Usually accompanied by a PFH.

BITE A surgical stitch. *Take a bigger bite* means "make the stitch longer."

BLACK CLOUD Bad luck that a medical student or resident brings along.

BLADE A surgeon, especially one who is dashing, bold, arrogant, and never in doubt (but often wrong).

BLAMESTORMING Assigning blame for mistakes, usually to the youngest and least-experienced doctor in sight.

BLEED 'EM To draw blood.

BLOODSUCKERS Those who are trained to draw blood samples, such as phlebotomists.

BLOWN Dilated (pupil).

BLOWN MIND Gunshot wound to the head.

BLUE BLOATER (OR BLUE BLOWER) Someone with chronic obstructive pulmonary disease (COPD), particularly someone with chronic bronchitis who has trouble inhaling.

BLUE PIPE A vein, as opposed to a red pipe, or artery.

BMT Bowel-Movement Taco (fecal matter trapped in female genitalia).

BMW Bitch, Moan, and Whine.

BOBBING FOR APPLES Using the finger to unclog a severely constipated patient.

BOHICA Bend Over, Here It Comes Again.

BONES AND GROANS A general hospital with no specialties.

BOOGIE A tumor.

BORDEAUX Urine with blood in it.

BOTTLE RETURN Removing a bottle lodged in the anal canal.

BOUGHT THE FARM Died.

BOUNCE BACK To readmit soon after discharge for the same or a related condition. A bounceback is a patient who has bounced back, as in "I admitted one of your bouncebacks last night."

BRAIN FRY Electroconvulsive therapy (ECT), used for depression.

BROTHEL SPROUTS Genital warts.

BROWN TROUT A stool that won't float—as opposed to an air biscuit, which does.

BSS Bilateral Samsonite Syndrome. Describes a patient admitted with both bags packed and expecting a long stay.

BTSOOM Beats The Shit Out Of Me.

BUFF 1. To rehash the patient's story to make it sound more appropriate for the patient to be referred (turfed) to another department. 2. To make sure all details regarding a patient's care are covered so that discharge or transfer to another service or facility will proceed smoothly and no excuses or objections can be raised to prevent the discharge or transfer—as in "Be sure to buff the guy in 702 before we send him to the nursing home."

BUFF 'EM UP To hydrate a patient and stabilize his or her electrolytes.

BUG JUICE Antibiotics.

BUGS IN THE RUG Pubic lice.

BULL IN THE RING A blocked large intestine.

BUNDY But Unfortunately Not Dead Yet.

BUNGEE JUMPER A patient who pulls on the catheter.

BUNNIES Sanitary napkins.

BUNNY BOILER A dangerously obsessive or unbalanced woman. From the film *Fatal Attraction.*

BURY THE HATCHET To accidentally leave a surgical instrument inside a patient.

BVA Breathing Valuable Air.

BWCO Baby Won't Come Out. Used when a caesarian section is needed to deliver the baby.

C & T WARD Cabbages and Turnips ward (coma ward).

CABBAGE Heart bypass surgery. From CABG, short for *coronary artery bypass graft*.

CALL BUTTON JOCKEY A patient who uses the call button all night long for no good reason.

CALLING DOCTOR BLUE (to specified location) Public address system code for "baffling case needing more doctors to take a look in the hope that one of them will know what to do."

CAMPERS Children with diseases, like cancer and diabetes, for which there are special summer camps.

CANCEL CHRISTMAS The patient is dying.

CAPTAIN KANGAROO Chief pediatrician, named for the former host of the pseudonymous children's television program.

CATH JOCKEY A cardiologist who catheterizes every patient he or she sees.

CBT Chronic Burger Toxicity (obesity).

CCFCCP Cuckoo For Cocoa Puffs (dementia or a similar condition). From the catchphrase originally used by Sonny, the Cocoa Puffs mascot, and later said of a woman on trial for murdering her husband as a means of describing her mental state.

CEILING SIGN Near levitation from the bed to the ceiling induced by an examination for abdominal tenderness.

CELESTIAL DISCHARGE Died, as in "Mr. Smith received a celestial discharge overnight."

CFT Chronic Food Toxicity (obesity).

CHAMPAGNE TAP A bloodless lumbar puncture.

CHANDELIER SIGN Near levitation when a patient who experiences extreme pain during a physical examination or cervical motion tenderness from a pelvic inflammation reacts to a touch by "jumping to the chandelier."

CHARTOMEGALY Having such frequent visits to the hospital that the patient has a large and growing chart.

CHEECH To give someone a patient with a bad problem that will require extensive testing and care, possibly beyond end of shift.

CHEERIOMA A particularly nasty tumor, one from which the patient will not recover. From *cheerio* meaning "good-bye."

CHOCOLATE HOSTAGE Used to describe constipation.

CHOLY, CHOLE A patient with cholecystitis (inflammation of the gallbladder).

CHROME-INDUCED ISCHEMIA A case of inexplicable chest pains that developed when the person was arrested and handcuffed.

CITY TAXI Used to describe the abuse of the free ride to the hospital provided in an ambulance.

CKS Cute Kid Syndrome.

CLL Chronic Low Life.

COCK DOC A urologist.

CODE AZURE A message to other staff to do nothing extraordinary to save a very ill patient who will die shortly no matter what is done.

CODE BROWN A bed full of excrement from an incontinent patient.

CODE YELLOW Urinary incontinence emergency.

COFFIN DODGER 1. Someone who survived against expectations. 2. A very old person.

COPD Chronic Old Person's Disease (unwell, with no specific cause).

CRAFT Can't Remember A Fucking Thing.

CRANIAL RECTOSIS Used to describe an idiot or an arrogant fool.

CRASH AND BURN A patient who is getting worse and needs to go to the ICU.

CREEPERS Geriatric patients using walkers and wheelchairs.

CRI Cranial-Rectal Insertion or Cranial-Rectal Inversion (head-up-ass syndrome).

CRINKLY A geriatric patient.

CRISPY CRITTER A patient with severe burns.

CROCK A hypochondriac.

CROP ROTATION Ambulance shuttle service from nursing home to surgery and back again.

CRS Can't Remember Shit.

CRT Can't Really Treat.

CRUMBLE (OR CRUMBLY) An elderly patient.

CRUMP To have a sudden change for the worse; to crash.

CTD Circling The Drain (close to death).

CTF Cletus The Fetus. Used to describe a baby born at twenty-three weeks or less, with poor survival prospects.

CTS Crazier Than Shit.

CUNTS AND RUNTS Maternity and pediatrics.

CUT AND PASTE To open a patient surgically, discover that there is no hope of a successful operation, and immediately sew the patient up.

CYA MEDICINE Cover Your Ass medicine (doing extra tests and documenting everything, especially with a litigious patient).

CYSTIC A child with cystic fibrosis.

D & D Divorced and Desperate. Used to describe a middle-aged woman who visits a doctor weekly just for male attention.

D & D'S Death and Doughnuts, the morbidity and mortality conferences (M & M's), where participants are served doughnuts and talk about patients who died.

DACB Drunk As Cooter Brown. A term referring to the legendary U.S. Civil War character who refused to join either army because he had family on both sides and chose chronic drunkenness as a solution.

DANCE The process of tying a surgical gown behind the surgeon's back, which involves a 180-degree spin by the surgeon. Example: "Shall we dance?"

DANDRUFF ON WHEELS Scabies or other transmissible flaky skin condition.

DBI Dirt Bag Index: the number of tattoos times the number of missing teeth equals the number of days since the patient last bathed.

DEAD SHOVEL A man who has a heart attack while shoveling snow.

DEEP FRY Radiation therapy.

DEMENT An Alzheimer's patient.

DEPARTURE LOUNGE A hospital's geriatric ward.

DFO 1. Done Fell Out (anything from fainting to cardiac arrest). 2. Drunk and Fell Over.

DIFFC Dropped In For a Friendly Chat (that is, the patient has no medical problem).

DIGGING FOR WORMS Surgery to remove varicose veins.

DIIK Damned If I Know.

DILF Doctor I'd Like to Fuck. Nursing slang for a good-looking doctor.

DIRT BAG A patient who enters the emergency room filthy and smelly. *See also* DBI.

DISCHARGED DOWNSTAIRS Transferred to the morgue.

DISHWASHER Sterilization machine.

DMFNFL Dumb Motherfucker Not Fit to Live.

DNK ("DINK") A patient who fails to keep an appointment.

DOC IN A BOX A small clinic or health center with ever-changing staff.

DOING THE TWIRLY Circling the drain (about to die).

DONOR CYCLES Motorcycles. Motorcyclists are the largest source of organ donations.

DOTTED Q *See* Q sign.

DOUBLE WHOPPER WITH CHEESE An obese female with genital thrush. The term derives from the name of the extra-large Burger King hamburger.

DOUGHNUT CT scanner. The term derives from its shape.

DOWN Used to refer to the length of time the heart stops in a case of cardiac arrest.

DPS 1. Droopy Penis Syndrome. Used to describe a patient wanting a Viagra prescription. 2. Disappearing Penis Syndrome. Used to describe the usual reaction of the male organ in response to the insertion of a catheter or an endoscope. 3. Dumb Parent Syndrome.

DQ Drama Queen.

DR. FEELGOOD A doctor who is indiscriminate about prescribing drugs.

DRINKECTOMY Separating a drunk from a can of beer (usually performed in the emergency room).

DROOLER A catatonic patient.

DROP A TUBE To insert a tube down someone's nose and esophagus into the stomach.

DRT Dead Right There (at the scene of the accident).

DRTTTT Dead Right There, There, There, and There (dead and in multiple parts at the scene of the accident).

DSB Drug-Seeking Behavior (faking illness to feed a narcotic addiction).

DSP Dumb Shit Profile.

DTMA Don't Transfer to Me Again.

DTS Danger To Shipping (a comment found in a particularly large patient's medical records).

DUCK A portable urinal for bedridden male hospital patients.

DUDE FACTOR A scoring factor based on social worth. An individual of questionable social worth who survives near-fatal injuries has a high dude factor. A professional person who slips in the bathroom and sustains a fatal injury has a low dude factor.

DUMP A bad, hard-to-dispose-of patient sent by another doctor; a patient no one seems to want.

DWPA Death/Dying With Paramedic Assistance.

EATING IN Intravenous feeding.

EATING THE BILL Providing care in the United States for indigent patients lacking insurance, as in "We ate the bill on that guy."

ECU Eternal Care Unit, as in "gone to the ECU" (dead).

EDGATWTTTF Elevator Doesn't Go All The Way To The Top Floor (stupid).

EMS Earn Money Sleeping (a joke at the expense of EMS [emergency medical services] responders).

EMT Extraordinary Masochistic Tendencies (a joke at the expense of emergency medical technicians).

ERNOBW Engine Running, No One Behind the Wheel (stupid).

EXPENSIVE CARE, EXPENSIVE SCARE Intensive care.

FABIANS Felt Awful But I'm All right Now Syndrome.

FAMILY CARE PLAN One child gets the sniffles, and the whole family gets a trip to the emergency room.

FANGER An oral surgeon.

FASCINOMA A fascinating tumor; any interesting malignancy. Implies that the tumor is not as interesting as the ensuing politics over who gets first authorship when the case is written up.

FD Fucking Drunk.

FDGB Fall Down, Go Boom.

FDSTW Found Dead, Stayed That Way.

FEATHER COUNT A measure of flakiness or wackiness in a patient, as in "He has a high feather count."

FEET-UP GENERAL A quiet rural hospital.

FERTILE MYRTLE A woman who gets pregnant repeatedly.

FFDID Found Face Down In Ditch.

FFDIG Found Face Down In Gutter.

FINE Fucked-up, Insecure, Neurotic, and Emotional.

FINGER WAVE A rectal examination.

FIRT Failed the Impact Resistance Test (car crash victim).

FITH Fucked In The Head (crazy).

FLAPPER A person with skin hanging in flaps due to serious injury.

FLB Funny Little Bumps (unexplained skin bumps).

FLEA A doctor specializing in internal medicine.

FLK Funny-Looking Kid (child who comes in and doesn't look quite right).

FLK W/GLM Funny-Looking Kid With a Good-Looking Mother.

FLKBCOTP Funny-Looking Kid, But Check Out The Parents.

FLOWER SIGN Flowers at the bedside. Indicates that the patient has a supportive family and might be a candidate for an early discharge.

FLP Funny-Looking Parent(s). Usually accompanied by an FLK.

FLUTTERING EYE SYNDROME Said of a patient faking unconsciousness.

FMPS Fluff My Pillow Syndrome. Said of a patient seeking attention and sympathy.

FOALS NEIGH Fuck Off And Let Someone Not Extremely Incompetent Get Here.

FODE Falling On Deaf Ears.

FOL, GOL, FOS Fat Old Lady, Gone Off Legs, Full Of Shit. Refers to a confused elderly woman unable to exercise at home who is now unable to move unaided and is badly constipated as a result.

FOOSH Fall Onto Outstretched Hand (as a cause of a broken wrist or arm).

FORD Found On Road Dead.

FOREVERECTOMY　A surgical procedure that lasts a very long time.

FOS　1. Found On Street. Describes an unidentified dead homeless person. 2. Full Of Shit (either physically or metaphorically constipated).

FPO　For Practice Only—that is, because the patient is FTD.

FREQUENT FLYER　Someone who is in and out of the emergency room, usually with minor complaints.

FREUD SQUAD　Psychiatrists.

FRIDAY CONSTRUCTION　Anatomical equivalent of cars made on Fridays, when workers' minds are more focused on the weekend than on the job at hand.

FRUIT SALAD　A group of stroke patients, all unable to take care of themselves.

FTD　Fixing To Die.

FTF　Failed To Fly (botched suicide).

FUBAR　Fucked Up Beyond All Recognition.

FUBIL　Fuck You, Buddy, I'm Leaving. Said by a doctor at a small hospital who is dumping a critically ill patient on a larger hospital on Friday afternoon before he or she leaves for the weekend.

FULL MOON　Full or overcrowded. Said of an emergency waiting room.

GACP　Gravity Assisted Concrete Poisoning. Said when someone jumped or fell from a great height.

GARDEN　Neurosurgical intensive-care ward, so called because of the "veggies" found there.

GARDENING　Attending to patients in neurological intensive care.

GAS 'EM　To do an arterial blood gas analysis.

GAS PASSER, GASSER　An anesthetist.

GDA　Gonna Die Anyway.

GENITAL HURTIES　Genital herpes.

GET BURNED　To make a mistake.

GGF Granny's Got a Fever (a workup of an elderly woman with a fever).

GLF Ground Level Fall (tripped and fell down).

GLM Good-Looking Mom.

GLORY ER Exciting emergency room cases.

GO DOWN THE TUBES To get sicker.

GO TO GROUND To fall out of a bed or a chair.

GOA Gone On Arrival (police turn up, ambulance turns up, fire brigade turns up, patient isn't there).

GOAT RODEO An emergency scene that goes badly (and resembles a bunch of people riding or wrestling goats).

GOD'S WAITING ROOM 1. Intensive-care unit. 2. Geriatric unit.

GOK God Only Knows.

GOLDBRICK A patient who demands more attention than a (minor) condition warrants.

GOLDEN ASS An affluent mother who treats the obstetrics nurses like servants.

GOMER Get Out of My Emergency Room. Extended to mean an elderly patient who is unable to communicate about his or her symptoms and is passed from one department to another.

GOMERGRAM An order for all available tests because the person is unable to explain what is wrong with him or her.

GONE CAMPING Said of a patient in an oxygen tent.

GOOBER Tumor. A roasted goober is a tumor after intensive radiation treatment; a healthy goober is a dead tumor patient ("The patient died, but the tumor survived").

GORILLACILLIN A very powerful antibiotic.

GORK 1. A patient on the way out; a hopeless case; someone who is brain dead. 2. God Only Really Knows.

GORKED Unresponsive and nonverbal, either because of sedation or because of a medical condition.

GORKED OUT Impaired mentally because of disease or substance abuse.

GPH Goddamns Per Hour.

GPO Good for Parts Only (won't survive).

GRAFOB Grim Reaper At the Foot Of the Bed (dying; dead).

GRANNY DUMPING Putting elderly relative in the emergency room, which often happens just before Christmas or a family holiday.

GRANNY FARM Nursing home or assisted living center, run by a granny farmer.

GRAPES Hemorrhoids.

GSW Gunshot wound.

GTHTTH Get The Hell To The Hospital. Used instead of *scoop and run* to indicate that a patient must be taken to the hospital immediately and deemed less alarming for the patient to hear.

GTO GOMER Tip Over (an elderly person injured from a trip or a fall).

GTTL Gone To The Light (died).

GUESSING TUBE A stethoscope.

HAIRY PSALMS Haven't Any Idea Regarding Your Patient; Send A Lot More Serum.

HALLUCINOMA A mass seen on a scan or X-ray that wasn't really there.

HALS Hit And Left Standing (apparently uninjured but in shock after a car accident).

HAMMER A local anesthetic.

HAMMERED Hit with numerous patients to admit while on duty. Example: "The night shift was hammered."

HAND THEM A BIBLE SO THEY CAN STUDY FOR THE FINAL The patient is about to die.

HANDBAG POSITIVE A confused patient (usually an elderly woman) lying on a hospital bed clutching a handbag.

HAPPY FEET A grand mal seizure.

HBD Had Been Drinking.

HEAD A brain-injury patient, as in "I've got a head to deal with."

HEAD BONK An otherwise uninjured patient who was struck on the head and went to the emergency room just to be sure nothing was wrong.

HEAD WHACK Head injury.

HEARTS AND FARTS Cardiology and geriatrics.

HEPATOLOGY CONFERENCE Doctors meeting at a pub or bar, as in "No late appointments. I'm going to a hepatology conference."

HEY, DOCS Alcoholics handcuffed to wheelchairs in big-city emergency rooms who shout "Hey, Doc!" when they see a white coat.

HI 5 HIV positive (*V* being the roman numeral for 5).

HIBGIA Had It Before, Got It Again.

HIGH-SERUM PORCELAIN LEVEL Said when a patient is malingering (more pointedly, is a crock of shit).

HIPPO 1. Hypochondriac. 2. Depressive.

HIT An admission to the hospital.

HIT AND RUN The act of operating quickly in order not to be late for another (usually nonmedical) appointment.

HIT HARD To get a lot of difficult patients in one shift.

HIVI Husband Is Village Idiot.

HMF Hysterical Mother Figure.

HOLE IN ONE A gunshot wound through the mouth or rectum.

HOPEFUL Hard-up Old Person Expecting Full Useful Life (not a priority patient for most hospitals).

HORRENDOPLASTY A difficult surgery with a prognosis that is probably poor.

HOSPITAL HOBO SYNDROME The tendency to visit multiple hospitals seeking attention or accommodation.

HOUSE RED Blood.

HTD Higher Than a Duck (from alcohol or drugs).

HTK Higher Than a Kite (from alcohol or drugs).

HTT Hot Tots and Twats (pediatrics and obstetrics-gynecology).

HURT ME AGAIN To get the victims of a train wreck or other disaster after just dealing with one set of disaster victims.

HVLP High-Velocity Lead Poisoning (gunshot wound).

"I FELL ON IT" Standard response from a patient asked how a foreign object found its way into the rectum.

ICING ON THE CAKE Lethal tumor discovered in the X-ray of a heart attack victim.

"IF YOU DIDN'T CHART IT, IT DIDN'T HAPPEN" Variant of *CYA medicine.*

IMPROVING HIS/HER CLAIM Said of the victim of a minor accident who needs no treatment but wants to support an insurance or legal claim.

INBREDS Doctors whose parents are also doctors.

INCARCEPHOBIA Fear of incarceration. Said of a hypochondriac prisoner who prefers the hospital to a jail cell.

INCARCERITIS Dubious illness acquired when arrested or in court.

INCIDENTALOMA Something found on a CT or other scan that requires action, even though it was not what the discoverer was looking for, as in "I found an incidentaloma in the adrenal gland." An incidentaloma is likely to be benign in nature but full of liability risks.

INCOMING SCUD An ambulance bringing victims of a train wreck or other disaster to the hospital.

INSURANCE PAIN Neck pain from an automobile accident secondary to minor damage to the car.

INSURANCE WHIPLASH Variant of *insurance pain.*

INTERNATIONAL HOUSE OF PANCAKES A neurology ward full of patients (usually stroke victims) babbling in different languages.

INTUBATE JUNIOR/WILLY To catheterize a penis (which often results in DPS—*see* definition 2).

IRREVERSIBLE Q Describes a tongue that keeps falling back out of the mouth despite repeated attempts to push it back in. Indicates a poor prognosis.

ISQ In Statu Quo. Often used during weekend surgical rounds, when no action is desirable and the patient's condition shows no change.

ITBNTL In The Box, Nail The Lid (dead or dying).

JAFFA Just Another Fat Fucking Administrator.

JAILITIS Dubious illness acquired while in custody or in a jail cell.

JLD Just Like Dad. Often used to explain an FLK.

JOURNAL OF ANECDOTAL MEDICINE A favorite (but unwritten) source of medical wisdom.

JPFROG Just Plain Fucking Ran Out of Gas (a death due to old age).

JPS Just Plain Stupid. Said of a self-induced injury involving lack of common sense.

KFO Knock the Fucker Out (to sedate a patient who is either obnoxious or screaming in pain).

KIDNEY STONE SQUIRM A spot (instant) diagnosis in an emergency.

KNIFE AND GUN CLUB An inner-city hospital that gets a lot of knife and gun wounds because of local street gangs or criminal groups. Example: "We have a very active knife and gun club, so the trauma department is busy."

KNIFE HAPPY Said of a surgeon too eager to operate.

KNUCKLEDRAGGER An orthopedic doctor or surgeon.

LAP Short for *laparoscopic,* as in *lap-chole* (laparoscopic cholecystectomy) and *lap-appy* (laparoscopic appendectomy).

LAST FLEA TO JUMP OFF A DEAD DOG Refers to oncologists (and sometimes other specialists) who don't seem to be able to let people die with dignity.

LEECHES Those who are trained to draw blood samples, such as phlebotomists.

LET'S GET OUT OF DODGE Let's finish the case.

LFTWM Looking For Three Wise Men. The term is applied to young pregnant females who deny having had intercourse.

LGFD Looks Good From the Doorway. Said of a patient no one wants to have anything to do with.

LIGNOCEPHALIC Wooden-headed (stupid or stubborn).

LIVER ROUNDS Friday-afternoon social event for attending doctors, residents, and medical students at which alcoholic beverages are served.

LMC Low Marble Count (low IQ).

LOBNH Lights On But Nobody Home (stupid; apparent awareness unsupported by intelligent response).

LOFD Looks Okay From the Door. Said of a patient no one wants to have anything to do with.

LOL Little Old Lady.

LOLFDGB Little Old Lady, Fall Down, Go Boom. Said of an elderly woman who fell down and hurt herself.

LOLINAD Little Old Lady In No Acute Distress.

LOLITS Little Old Lady In Tennis Shoes.

LOOP THE LOOP Flamboyant surgical rearrangement of the intestines.

LOOSE CHANGE A dangling limb in need of amputation.

LPT Low Pain Threshold.

LRO Luck Ran Out. Said of a patient who cheated death before, but not this time.

LWS Low Wallet Syndrome. Refers to poor patients in the United States without insurance.

M & M'S Morbidity and mortality conferences, where the ER doctors, residents, medical students, pathologists, and other specialists gather to discuss past cases in which there was an error or the patient did not do as well as expected. The conferences are usually held once a week in the early morning. Residents have to present the cases and are fair game for the audience of Monday-morning quarterbacks.

M SIGN Said of a patient who just says "Mmmm."

MARPS Mind Altering Recreational Pharmaceuticals (recreational drugs).

MARRIAGEABLE MONSTER A young female patient who has successfully undergone major plastic surgery.

MATERN-A-TAXI An ambulance taken when a pregnant woman has called for it because her contractions come every two minutes, but then she doesn't have a single contraction during a thirty-minute trip to the hospital.

MCBP Member of the College of Bystander Physicians (a doctor having a look at a patient just out of curiosity).

MEAL Doctors' rounds of gastrointestinal patients. Example: "Dr. Smith is having a meal."

MEAT HOOKS Surgical instruments.

METABOLIC CLINIC The staff cafeteria.

METH MOUTH A finding (usually advanced tooth decay) in a patient severely addicted to methamphetamine.

MFB, CFD Measure For Box, Call For Dirt (severely ill or nearly dead).

MFI Motherfucking Infarction (a very large myocardial infarction; a major heart attack).

MGM SYNDROME Said of a patient who is faking an illness or an injury but putting on a really good show.

MIDI Myocardial Infarction During Intercourse (heart attack during sex).

MILF Mother I'd Like to Fuck.

MOBILE DRIP STANDS Fire department personnel (often found at accidents and other emergency situations alongside paramedics).

MOLAR MASHER A dentist.

MU PAIN Made-Up pain. Used to describe patients reporting imaginary maladies who request sick notes for employers or for insurance claims.

MUH Messed-Up Heart.

MUTUAL OF SACRAMENT Medicare.

N = 1 TRIAL A polite term for experimenting on a patient, as opposed to doing a formal experiment with a greater number (N) of subjects.

NAD Not Actually Done.

NARS Not A Rocket Scientist (low IQ).

NEGATIVE WALLET BIOPSY After confirmation of financial status, transfer of a patient to a cheaper hospital because she or he has no health insurance or money.

NETMA Nobody Ever Tells Me Anything (generally a doctor's gripe entered on a patient's chart).

NEUROFECAL SYNDROME Having shit for brains.

NGMI Not Going to Make It.

NKDA Not Known, Didn't Ask.

NLPR No Longer Playing Records (dying).

NOT EVEN IN THE BALL GAME Confused and senile.

NPS New Parent Syndrome (excitable, nervous, worried).

NQR Not Quite Right.

NQRITH Not Quite Right In The Head.

NSA Nonstandard Appearance (what an FLK grows into).

O SIGN Used to describe a comatose patient with mouth agape.

OAP Overanxious Patient.

OBE Open at Both Ends (diarrhea and vomiting).

OBS   Obvious Bullshit.

OBS AND GOBS   Obstetrics and gynecology.

OFIG   One Foot In the Grave.

OFIGATOOS   One Foot In the Grave And The Other One Slipping.

OH-NO SECOND   The time from making an error (for example, dropping that hard-to-get blood sample immediately after obtaining it) to saying "Oh, no!"

OLD PERSON'S FRIEND   Pneumonia, which often carries off elderly patients.

OLD TROUT   A patient who is old but quick-witted.

OLIGONEURONAL   Having few brain cells (stupid).

OMGWTFBBQ   Oh, My God, a What-The-Fuck Barbecue (a person mangled or burned in a fire or car crash).

OOH-AAHS   Those who gather to gawk and exclaim at an accident scene or other disaster.

OPD   Obnoxious Personality Disorder.

ORGAN RECITAL   A hypochondriac's medical history.

ORTHOPOD   An orthopedist.

OSTEOCEPHALIC   Boneheaded (stupid).

OSTRICH TREATMENT   Pretending it's not there and hoping it goes away.

OTD & DTR   Out The Door and Down The Road (discharged).

OTDPDS   Out The Door Pretty Damn Soon (scheduled for discharge).

OVERPRICED CARPENTER   An orthopedist.

P4P   Penicillin For Prick (given for penile discharge).

PAFO   Pissed (drunk) And Fell Over.

PANINVESTIGRAM   An order for all the tests when the patient complains of pain and no one knows what's causing it.

PARENTECTOMY Removing parents as an effective cure for a child's problems.

PATHOLOGY OUTPATIENTS Follow-up for dead people.

PAWS UP Dead.

PBAB Pine Box At Bedside (dying).

PBOO Pine Box On Order (dying).

PBS Pretty Bad Shape.

PECKER CHECKER 1. A urologist. 2. A doctor of sexual diseases. 3. Navy slang for the ship's doctor.

PEDIATRON A pediatrician.

PEEK AND SHRIEK To open a patient surgically, discover an incurable condition, and close the incision immediately.

PEFYC Pre-Extricated For Your Convenience. Said of a traffic accident victim who has gone through a windshield.

PERCUSSIVE MAINTENANCE The sharp tap or bang that cures faulty equipment.

PERF To perforate; to burst.

PFH Parent(s) From Hell (custodians of a BFH—*see* definition 3).

PGT Pissed (drunk) and Got Thumped.

PHARMACEUTICALLY ENHANCED PERSONALITY Stoned or medicated.

PHAT Pretty Hot And Tempting. Said as a warning to others.

PIA Pain In the Ass.

PID Pus In Dere, where *dere* is a mispronounced "there" (pelvic inflammatory disease, which has the acronym PID).

PID SHUFFLE The walk of a patient with pelvic inflammatory disease (the patient hunches over, clutching the abdomen, and shuffles along with legs wide apart).

PILLOW THERAPY Describes the urge to smother an annoying patient.

PIMP To ask a medical student or resident difficult questions.

PINK PUFFER A patient breathing rapidly because of lung disease.

PINKY CHEATER A latex finger-cover used in gynecological and proctological examinations.

PIT Emergency room.

PIT HER To give a pregnant woman Pitocin to induce labor.

PLANK POSITIVE Stupid, as in "thick as a plank."

PLAYER A complaining, irritating patient.

PLH Pray Long and Hard. Said when a patient is in danger of dying.

PLTDP Practice Limited To Dead People. Said of doctors who would continue to treat, even when there are no signs of life. Example: "He would treat on the way to the morgue."

PNEUMOCEPHALIC Airheaded (stupid).

PNR Person Needed a Ride (a patient had a minor ailment but called an ambulance instead of a taxi).

PODO-ORAL Foot-in-mouth. Rarely used *by* senior staff but sometimes used *about* them.

POLICEMAN LESION A lesion on an X-ray so obvious that a police officer would spot it.

POPTA Passed Out Prior To Arrival.

PORCELAIN-LEVEL TEST A fictitious blood test ordered to communicate to a colleague that the patient is malingering (more pointedly, is a crock of shit).

PORG Person Of Restricted/Retarded Growth (a small person).

POSITIVE HILTON SIGN 1. Refers to a demanding patient who expects Hilton Hotel luxury. 2. Indicates a patient well enough to leave.

POST-WEEKEND FATIGUE SYNDROME An ailment common during Monday-morning rounds.

POTTED PLANT A person in a persistent vegetative state.

POX DOCS Doctors who work in clinics specializing in sexually transmitted diseases.

PPA Practicing Professional Alcoholic.

PPP Piss-Poor Protoplasm (a dismal specimen of humanity).

PPPP Particularly Piss-Poor Protoplasm (A patient who is unlikely to survive).

PRATFO Patient Reassured And Told to Fuck Off.

PRE-DETENTION STRESS DISORDER The condition of a person who fakes medical symptoms when the police put on handcuffs.

PREEMIE A premature infant.

PRE-STIFF A terminally comatose patient.

PSYCODE Code Blue in a psychiatric hospital, usually called because a patient has passed out from the side effects of medication.

PUMPKIN POSITIVE Lacking in intelligence—that is, the brain is so small that a penlight shone into the patient's mouth or ear would light up the whole head like a Halloween pumpkin.

(CODE) PURPLE A call to paramedics to attend a dead body.

(CODE) PURPLE PLUS A call to paramedics to attend a dead body that has started to fester.

PVC CHALLENGE Intubation. PVC is the plastic material used to make the inserted tube.

PWT Po' (poor) White Trash (someone with a medical condition related to his or her supposed lifestyle).

Q SIGN Refers to a patient who is unconscious, perhaps terminally ill, with the mouth open and the tongue hanging out. *Dotted Q* means that flies are landing on the tongue (the person is dying or dead).

Q-TIP Elderly person (with white hair).

QUACKPRACTOR A chiropractor.

QWERTYITIS What doctors suffer from when they spend more time on a computer than with actual patients. Refers to the top row of letters on a keyboard: q-w-e-r-t-y(-u-i-o-p).

RAINBOW DRAW Taking a full vial of blood for a tube of every color available when a doctor's blood-draw orders are illegible.

RAISIN FARM Geriatric ward, nursing home, or assisted living center, run by a raisin farmer.

RALPHIE MCYAKKERS Young drunks vomiting.

RAPID LEAD INFUSION Solution for an obnoxious patient who ought to be shot.

RBG Received By God (dead, complete with a receipt for admission to heaven).

RBS Really Bad Shape.

REAR ADMIRAL A proctologist.

RED PIPE An artery, as opposed to a blue pipe, or vein.

REEKER A smelly patient.

RETROSPECTOSCOPE Instrument of hindsight.

REVERSIBLE Q SIGN Describes being able to push a patient's tongue back into the mouth to form the O sign.

ROAD CHILI, ROAD PIZZA Driver, motorcyclist, or passenger ejected and splattered in a car accident.

ROAD MAP Injuries from going through a car windshield face first.

ROAD RASH Abrasions seen on car accident victims who fell on asphalt or were dragged on it.

ROCKET ROOM A ward or unit where there are many deaths (many transfers to the ECU, or eternal care unit).

ROOTERS Indigents and hangers-on who gather in big-city emergency rooms to be entertained by legitimate cases.

ROUNDING UP THE USUAL SUSPECTS Ordering a full round of tests for a given set of symptoms.

RT Room Temperature (dead).

RTT WITH A BBB Rat-a-Tat-Tat with a Baseball Bat (hit with a blunt instrument).

RUDY BAGA A patient with terminal brain injury or in a persistent vegetative state (after rutabaga, the vegetable).

RULE OF FIVE If more than five of the patient's orifices are obscured by tubing, the patient has no chance of surviving.

SADDLES Sanitary napkins (towels) for women in the maternity ward, so called for their size and the bowlegged effect of wearing them.

SAS Sick As Shit.

SBI Something Bad Inside (undiagnosed cancer or unexpected serious condition found when performing surgery).

SBLEO (PRONOUNCED "S-B-LEO") Suicide By Law Enforcement Officer.

SBOD Stupid Bitch/Bastard On Drugs.

SCOOP AND RUN To transport immediately to the nearest hospital. The opposite of *stay and play*.

SCRATCH AND SNIFF A gynecological examination.

SCREAMIN' MIGHTY JESUS Spinal meningitis.

SCUT WORK Routine, often menial work like drawing blood and filling out lab slips.

SEIZER A child with epilepsy.

SEND FOR LABS To draw blood and send the specimens for analysis.

SEND HIM/HER REDLINE To send him/her directly and urgently (to a specified location).

SERUM PORCELAIN A battery of blood tests performed on an elderly patient. The reference to a toilet bowl ("porcelain") suggests a waste of time and resources.

SF SCALE Sphincter Factor scale (a one to ten scale indicating the degree of bowel-loosening in response to an emergency).

SFS Stinky Foot Syndrome (often associated with homeless people).

SHA Ship His Ass. Said when patients refuse to be discharged.

SHAD Syphilitic, Hypochondriac, Alcoholic, Degenerate.

SHADOW GAZER A radiologist.

SHANDY TAP A bloodless lumbar puncture.

SHITS & SPITS A·lab technician's term for a patient's stool and sputum samples; also, the instruction to obtain these samples.

SHORT-ORDER CHEF A morgue worker.

SHOTGUN LABS To order many lab tests, hoping that one will be abnormal and therefore provide a clue as to what's wrong with the patient. Some patients may require *shotgunning*.

SHPOS Subhuman Piece Of Shit.

SHS Sullen, Hostile, Stupid. Often used to describe an inner-city drug or alcohol addict.

SICK Very sick and near death.

SICKLER A child with sickle-cell anemia.

SIDEWALK SOUFFLÉ A person who has fallen or jumped from a building onto the sidewalk.

SIEVE A doctor who admits almost every patient she or he sees.

SILVER BRACELET AWARD Used to describe a patient brought in wearing handcuffs.

SILVER GOOSE, SILVER STALLION A proctoscope.

SIO Sleeping It Off.

SKEPTICEMIA A condition suffered by two doctors debating which therapy to implement.

SLAMMED Hit very hard.

SLASHERS General surgeons.

SLMF YOYO So Long, Motherfucker, You're On Your Own. *See* AMYOYO.

SLOUGH A patient inappropriately or unfairly unloaded from one hospital unit to another.

SLOW CODE Usually designates an elderly patient who is very ill but wants everything done to preserve life although everyone on the medical team disagrees with the value of taking such measures. "Mr. Smith is a slow code" means "Don't run to get the crash cart. Take your time."

SMASHOLA A patient with multiple blunt trauma injuries, usually resulting from a car accident.

SMELLY BRIDGE The area between the anus and the back of the scrotum; the perineum.

SMELT *See* they're going to box like smelt.

SMILING MIGHTY JESUS Spinal meningitis.

SMURF SIGN A patient who is blue or going blue (cyanotic). Smurfs are sky-blue cartoon figures.

SNOW To accidentally give a patient too much medication, or to mix medications, so that a patient goes into an altered state of consciousness. Example: "Don't snow that patient with drug X and drug Y at the same time."

SNOWED Being in a state of altered consciousness because of too much medication or mixed medications.

SNUD Sick Nigh Unto Death.

SOB Shortness Of Breath.

SOCMOB Standing On a Corner Minding one's Own Business (when inexplicably injured).

SODDI Some Other Doctor Did It. Said when one doctor's botched job must be corrected by another.

SOFA SURFER A homeless person who sleeps on friends' sofas and floors and ends up in the emergency room when he or she has nowhere else to stay.

SOFT ADMISSION An admission to the hospital that only a sieve would accept.

SOLDIERS Children with chronic gastrointestinal diseases, like Crohn's disease.

SPARK 'EM To defibrillate a patient.

SPECIAL K *See* vitamin K.

SPEED BUMPS Hemorrhoids.

SPOTS AND DOTS The traditional set of childhood diseases: measles, mumps, and chicken pox.

SQUASH The brain.

SQUIRREL An eccentric (squirrelly) or hypochondriac patient who can make life difficult. From the motivational phrase "Squirrels get sick, too," said to remind staff that even hypochondriacs may have real medical problems.

SRI Something Wrong Inside (undiagnosable problem).

SSDD Same Shit, Different Day, often used for a frequent flyer.

ST. ELSEWHERE Derisive term for any nonteaching hospital.

STAGE MOTHER A woman accompanying the patient who encourages the patient to exaggerate the complaint, often to obtain a particular diagnosis or to get an unnecessary prescription.

STAMP A skin graft.

STAY AND PLAY To treat a patient at the site of an accident. The opposite of *scoop and run.*

STOOL MAGNET A resident doctor who always seems to get very sick patients with complicated symptoms.

STREAM TEAM Collectively, the urology department.

STUPIDITY PANEL A lab test for patient stupidity that, when invented, will earn its inventor a fortune.

SUMMER TEETH Used to describe a patient with missing teeth: "Some are there and some aren't."

SUPRATENTORIAL "Above the tentorium," loosely meaning "in the brain cortex," used to imply that something is all in a patient's head, imaginary. Example: "This patient's condition is supratentorial."

SVRI Something Very Wrong Inside (usually terminal).

SWAG Scientific Wild-Ass Guess.

SWEET MILK Propofol, a short-acting intravenous anesthetic.

SWI Something Wrong Inside.

SWW Sick, Wet, and Whiny. Normally refers to an infant.

SYB Save Your Breath. Said of patients who don't take advice.

T & T SIGN Tattoo and Tooth sign. An indicator of survival: those who are tattooed and toothless are likely to survive major injuries.

TAINT SPOT The perineum; the area between the anus and the scrotum. "It ain't this and it ain't that."

TANK 'EM UP To give a patient who is dehydrated a lot of fluid.

TASH TEST An observation that a patient may have HIV (because he has a Freddie Mercury–like moustache).

TATT, TAT 1. Talks All The Time. 2. Tired All The Time.

TATTOO TITER A way to measure the likelihood that a patient is insane. The more tattoos the patient has, the higher the probability of mental illness.

TATTOO-TO-TOOTH RATIO (TTR) A rough measure of social class. A higher ratio supposedly indicates a higher likelihood of experiencing trauma, as well as an increased likelihood of surviving said trauma.

TAX SUCKER Someone who does not need an ambulance but calls anyway because it's free.

TAXIDERMY CONSULT A call to consult a taxidermist (the patient is about to die).

TBC Total Body Crunch (multiple injuries).

TBP Total Body Pain.

TDS Terminal Deceleration Syndrome. Used to describe death by car accident, jumping, or having a parachute fail to open.

TEC Transfer to Eternal Care (dead).

TEETH Tried Everything Else. Try Homeopathy.

TF BUNDY Totally Fucked But Unfortunately Not Dead Yet.

TFO Too Fucking Old (used to describe a person dying of old age).

TFTB Too Fat To Breathe.

THC Three Hots (hot meals) and a Cot. Used to describe what the local homeless seek in the emergency room.

THERAPEUTIC MONITORING Monitoring a patient because it makes the doctor feel better.

THEY'RE GOING TO BOX LIKE SMELT The patients are going to die.

THORAZINE SHUFFLE The slow, lumbering gait of psychiatric patients dosed with phenothiazines (tranquilizers and antipsychotics).

THREE-TOED SLOTH A patient with diminished capacities, usually from long-term alcoholism.

THROCKMORTON'S SIGN When a penis is visible on an X-ray, tradition holds that it will point to the side of the body where an abnormal condition will be present.

TLC Tube, Lavage, and Charcoal (given to a poisoning victim).

TMB Too Many Birthdays. Said of a person dying of old age.

TMI Three Meaningless Initials, as in John Smith, TMI. Applied to doctors with qualifications rather than ability.

TOASTER Defibrillator.

TOBP Tired of Being Pregnant. Usually said of a patient demanding a caesarian.

TONTINE TREATMENT Said when there is an urge to put a pillow over the face of an irritating patient. Alludes to a type of will called a tontine.

TORTURE ME Variant of *hurt me again*.

TORTURE ROOM Intensive-care unit (because of the number of invasive tubes, monitors, and experimental treatments found there).

TOUGH STICK A patient who is difficult to draw blood from.

TOXIC CONFUSIONAL STATE The condition of a confused, usually elderly person whose confusion is due to constipation and the attendant toxic buildup in the body.

TRAIN WRECK A patient with multiple problems and complications who will keep staff up all night.

TRAUMA GODS Deities whom emergency staff jokingly blame for major emergencies.

TRAUMA HANDSHAKE Digital rectal examination (every major trauma patient gets one).

TREAT AND STREET To treat a patient in the emergency room or a clinic without admitting the patient to the hospital.

TRIGGER-HAPPY A doctor who gives an injection for everything.

TRO Time Ran Out.

TSL Too Stupid to Live.

TSS Toxic Sock Syndrome. Often refers to a homeless person.

TTFO Told To Fuck Off.

TTOAST Take Them Out And Shoot Them.

TTR *See* tattoo-to-tooth ratio.

TUBE Totally Unnecessary Breast Exam.

TURF (OUT) 1. To send a patient to another department in the hospital. 2. To get rid of a patient by referring the patient to another medical team.

TURN AND BASTE To care for an incontinent patient; to roll over and clean up a patient after a Code Brown.

TWA Third World Assassins. Derisive term for the allegedly poor medical care delivered by doctors who went to medical schools in foreign countries.

TWITCH A hypochondriac.

TWO BEERS The number of beers every patient involved in an alcohol-related car accident claims to have consumed before the accident.

TWO DUDES The usual answer when a doctor asks a male patient who beat him up, as in "I was walking down the street minding my own business when these two dudes jumped me for no reason." The implication is that the patient would have won the fight against only one dude.

TWSAM Trash Will Survive And Multiply.

UBI Unexplained Beer Injury.

UDI Unidentified Drinking Injury.

UFO Unidentified Frozen Object (unidentified dead homeless person in the winter).

UNCLEAR MEDICINE Nuclear medicine.

UNDERDOSE An overdose that doesn't kill the patient.

UNIVAC Unusually Nasty Infection, Vultures Are Circling.

UPF Unpassed Fart (a gaseous distended abdomen).

URBAN OUTDOORSMAN A homeless man.

VAC Vultures Are Circling (the patient is dying).

VAMPIRES Those who take blood samples.

VBT Very Bad Thing.

VD Veak and Dizzy. Used to describe an older person feeling vaguely unwell who shows up at the emergency room at 2:00 AM complaining of feeling "weak and dizzy." VD more commonly stands for "venereal disease."

VEGETABLE GARDEN Coma ward.

VEGGIE A patient requiring intensive care; a patient incapable of movement.

VELCRO Family or friends who accompany a patient everywhere.

VERY CLOSE VEINS Varicose veins.

VIAGGRAVATION What a doctor gets from a patient who insistently demands erectile dysfunction medication.

VIP Very Intoxicated Person.

VITAMIN H Haldol, a tranquilizer given to combative people.

VITAMIN K Ketamine, a powerful injectable anesthetic chiefly used on animals but also a common street drug. When smoked or snorted, it can cause hallucinations. Also called Special K.

VITAMIN L Lasix, to treat high blood pressure.

VITAMIN M Morphine.

VITAMIN P A diuretic given to increase urine flow.

VITAMIN V 1. Diazepam (Valium, Valrelease), commonly used to treat anxiety and insomnia. 2. Valium or other sedative given intravenously.

VOMIT Victim Of Modern Imaging Technology. Used to suggest treating the patient, not the report from radiology, particularly in reference to invasive procedures for false positives.

VTMK Voice To Melt Knickers (the sexy voice deliberately cultivated by some doctors).

WADAO Weak And Dizzy All Over.

WALKING TIME BOMB Someone with a condition that could be fatal at any moment, such as an aortic aneurysm.

WALL A doctor who resists admitting patients—the opposite of a sieve.

WALLET BIOPSY A check by the hospital before treatment to confirm that a patient is insurance-qualified.

WARD X The morgue.

WEED PULLER An obstetrician.

WHEEZER An asthmatic.

WHITE CLOUD Used to describe a doctor who tends to have uneventful on-call nights. Example: "Dr. Smith has a white cloud. She had only one admit last night." *See also* black cloud.

WHITE MICE Tampons.

WIG PICKER A therapist or psychologist.

WIN THE GAME To discharge all of the patients for which a doctor is responsible, so that he or she will have no ward rounds coming up. Example: "Mike won the game and doesn't have to round this weekend." The win is also called a Yahtzee after the popular dice game.

WITCH DOCTOR A doctor specializing in internal medicine.

WNL 1. Within Normal Limits. 2. We Never Looked. Said to joke about oversights. 3. Will Not Listen. Said of a patient who won't take medical advice.

WOFTAM (**PRONOUNCED** "**WOFF-TAM**") Waste Of Fucking Time And Money.

WOGS Wrath Of God Syndrome (visited upon junior doctors by more senior staff).

WRINKLY Geriatric.

WWI Walked While Intoxicated (and fell over).

YAVIS Young, Attractive, Verbal, Intelligent, Successful.

YMRASU Your Medical Records Are Screwed Up.

YOYO You're On Your Own. 1. Refers to a patient who signs out against advice. 2. What one doctor says to another about a problem case that is completely baffling. *See also* AMYOYO; SLMF YOYO.

ZEBRA A strange or unexpected disease. From the saying "When you hear hoofbeats, the smart money is on horses, not zebras."

Recommended Resources

Books

Bed Number Ten by Sue Baier and Mary Zimmeth Schomaker (Boca Raton, FL: CRC Press, 1986) Paralyzed by Guillain-Barré syndrome, a Houston housewife, Sue Baier, spent eleven months in a hospital as family and friends rallied to ease her fear of a health-care system that seemed indifferent to her suffering and reduced her to feeling like an annoyance. Although the book is more than twenty years old, it is still sadly reflective of the practice of medicine in many hospitals.

Bloodletting and Miraculous Cures by Vincent Lam (Toronto: Anchor Canada, 2006) This award-winning debut novel about daily life in an ER purports to be fiction, but Lam actually practices as an emergency doctor in a major urban hospital, and his day job obviously energizes the book's twelve interwoven stories. Medical students take note—fallibility rules, and it stings.

Complications: A Surgeon's Notes on an Imperfect Science (New York: Metropolitan Books, 2002) and *Better: A Surgeon's Notes on Performance* (New York: Metropolitan Books, 2007), both by Atul Gawande, M.D. In these books, Gawande topples the assumption that all surgeons are arrogant and aloof, humanizing the profession with soaring prose and self-deprecating humor.

How Doctors Think by Jerome Groopman, M.D. (Boston: Houghton Mifflin, 2007) Wise and compassionate insights into the complex diagnostic process by a prominent doctor and journalist (*The New Yorker*) who believes that the best kind of medical practice is a "mix of science and soul."

Mayo Clinic Family Health Book edited by Scott C. Litin, M.D. (New York: HarperResource, 2003) First published in 1990 and now in a third edi-

319

tion, this hefty (seven pounds) reference manual covers a wide variety of medical issues in its 1,424 pages, with tips for care of the newborn and the elderly and everyone in between. Carefully positioned by Mayo Clinic experts as an ally for healthy living rather than a self-diagnosis tool, the book also has a useful first-aid section that covers crises as simple as a cut and as scary as choking.

Through the Patient's Eyes: Understanding and Promoting Patient-Centered Care edited by Margaret Gerteis, Susan Edgman-Levitan, Jennifer Daley, and Thomas L. Delbanco (Hoboken, NJ: Jossey-Bass, 1993) Informally dubbed the "Picker playbook" because it picks up on Harvey Picker's original vision for patient-centered care and adds solid, research-based advice, this book is intended for hospital insiders but would also be useful for anyone who wants to know how hospitals can make life better for patients and their families. While communication and compassion are key themes throughout, the book starts with the recommendation that each patient should be treated as an individual with unique needs. What a concept!

An Uncertain Inheritance: Writers on Caring for Family edited by Nell Casey (New York: William Morrow/HarperCollins, 2007) Often overworked and underappreciated, family caregivers are seldom ready for the stress and fatigue that go with the challenge of dealing with an ill or dying loved one. Nineteen contributors (including Dr. Jerome Groopman; see *How Doctors Think,* above) share their experiences of anger, grief, frustration, and loneliness.

Webster's New World Medical Dictionary (Hoboken, NJ: Wiley, 2008) The third edition of a best-seller, with more than 8,500 definitions, all vetted by doctors and all organized for quick and easy reference. There is also a useful appendix on vitamins and popular medications.

Web Sites

It has been estimated that more than 100,000 Web sites deal with health-related issues. A lot dispense misleading or outdated information, and a lot offer sage advice based on data that are frequently reviewed and refreshed. Does any single Web site have a lock on accuracy? No. But the following recommendations come close—especially those offering medical information and advice. Most have earned their credibility, and many are consulted by medical professionals themselves. But browse with caution and avoid self-diagnosing. Instead, use the sites below to arm yourself with smart questions for your own doctor. And beware the phrase "possible causes," often used to flag the potential (but not yet proven) triggers of a condition or illness. You might be tempted to leap to a scary assumption based on inconclusive evidence—and that could make you sick.

All of the following Web addresses were valid at the time of writing. Some sites may have since moved or changed their names. Others may have been shut down. If you receive something like a "page not found" response when you enter an address in your browser, try using your favorite search engine to go on a hunt for key terms in the description.

Organizations Committed to Improving Patient and Family Experiences

Institute for Family-Centered Care (www.familycenteredcare.org) Bev Johnson leads this passionate nonprofit organization that is dedicated to integrating patients and their families into hospital-care partnerships. Once primarily involved with neonatal and children's hospitals, the organization has expanded its mission in recent years to include adult facilities.

Institute for Healthcare Improvement (www.ihi.org) Safety, effectiveness, patient-centeredness, timeliness, efficiency, equity—these are the goals of this nonprofit group out to change the quality of health-care delivery globally. Based in Cambridge, Massachusetts, and led by the noted pediatrician and Harvard professor Don Berwick, IHI has recruited some of the field's smartest thinkers to its team.

NRC Picker (www.nrcpicker.com) The late Harvey Picker's original vision for patient-centered care has morphed into a for-profit corporation that measures patient satisfaction and provides the tools to improve performance scores. The organization hosts an annual international symposium that gathers leading health-care voices from all over the world.

Planetree (www.planetree.org) Planetree is a Connecticut-based nonprofit organization that specializes in the how-to of delivering patient- and family-centered care using the accumulated wisdom from hundreds of focus groups conducted around the world. It stresses treating the patient's family and friends as partners in care.

Picker Institute (www.pickerinstitute.org) Perhaps because Harvey Picker wanted his advocacy of patient-centered care to be untainted by profit motives, he distanced himself from NRC Picker (see above) some years ago and then led the charge into England, Germany, and Switzerland from the nonprofit institute's Maine office. The Web site is worth a look for its European perspective and for proof that patients complain in a universal language.

Press Ganey (www.pressganey.com) Among the organizations devoted to the mission of happier patients and families, this is the big one. It claims that 40 percent of U.S. hospitals use its services and programs to improve their quality of care.

General Health Information

Canadian Institute for Health Information (http://secure.cihi.ca/) CIHI is an independent nonprofit organization that tracks health issues across Canada, reporting the results of various studies and surveys. Because it addresses themes like costs and wait-times that challenge patients and providers everywhere, the information provided is universally interesting. Check out the encouraging results of a nursing job-satisfaction survey.

Centers for Disease Control and Prevention (www.cdc.gov) A global authority once consulted chiefly by medical professionals tracking outbreaks of various alarming epidemics, the CDC now welcomes to its Web site anyone with an interest in preventing illness and injury.

Health Canada (www.hc-sc.gc.ca) Somewhat limited and occasionally marked by political grandstanding, the Canadian government's official health site nonetheless offers solid information on a variety of topics. Just don't look for cutting-edge answers. This is health lite.

Mayo Clinic (www.mayoclinic.com) The Web site of this world-famous medical facility now offers "tools for healthier lives," and they are organized superbly here, including quick links to sixteen Healthy Living Centers that range in theme from Baby's Health to Working Life. The senior editors are all Mayo Clinic physicians and educators. The site's message appears to be "Stay healthy so you won't need us."

MedicineNet.com (www.medicinenet.com) Produced by a network of more than seventy physicians certified by the American Board of Medical Specialties, this Web site, part of the WebMD network, has a breezy and eclectic tone, but the information is grounded in solid medical principles. In the wide-ranging articles, readers can learn how to identify anything from the signs of a stroke to the "six sex mistakes men make." The latter article contains advice for men who take all their erotic cues from popular movies or literature. Duh.

MedlinePlus (http://medlineplus.gov) A service of the U.S. National Library of Medicine (the world's largest medical library) and the National Institutes of Health, this Web site is a massive one-stop resource with answers to just about any health question ever asked. Consulted regularly by health professionals, the site may initially daunt the average consumer, but the information is surprisingly accessible, and answers are easy to understand.

National Institutes of Health (http://health.nih.gov) Learn why that constant tingle in your wrist could be carpal tunnel syndrome or why you experience stress when your spouse doesn't—or if there's any cure for that rare and dangerous disease you've never heard of. Health topics are alphabetized for speedy access, and the tone throughout is sober but friendly. The Web site is linked to other accredited resources for deeper digging.

PubMed (www.ncbi.nlm.nih.gov) Consider this Web site of the National Center for Biotechnology Medicine a vast library, packed with esoteric information that initially appears to be of interest only to medical researchers. But scroll down the opening page to the PubMed Central tab, and a mouse click will take you to a search engine for virtually every professional journal article ever written about a drug, a disease, a condition, or an issue. That's where it gets really interesting.

Revolution Health (www.revolutionhealth.com) With educational articles provided by the likes of Mayo Clinic and Harvard University and with editorial supervision by physicians, the site is both credible and friendly. Here you'll find advice on soothing sunburned skin right next to helpful information about the signs and symptoms of a brain tumor, and that mix may be somewhat confusing until you realize that Revolution Health has positioned itself at the center of a large virtual community with links to all kinds of nonclinical help. It calls itself a consumer-centric health company.

WebMD (www.webmd.com) Find a doctor. Find a hospital. Find a drug and then read user reviews. Find a support group. Overseen by an independent medical review board composed of four physicians, the site is community driven and encourages members to share their experiences. Also included are a handy Symptom Checker for a variety of common conditions and A to Z Health Guides, including a first-aid reference with excellent advice that also cautions anyone in doubt to immediately call 911.

Emergency Care

eMedicine (www.emedicine.com/emerg) Universally respected, this Web site bills itself as "The Continually Updated Clinical Reference." It is a goldmine of professional articles about all the conditions that send people to the emergency room and how to treat them. The site is edited by physicians and sponsored by WebMD.

Madness: Tales of an Emergency Room Nurse (http://emergency-room-nurse .blogspot.com) A blog with occasionally cranky ruminations about daily life in the emergency room by a veteran nurse who seems to spend her shifts shaking her head over the infinite human capacity for stupid behavior. Not for those with a sentimental view of nursing but nonetheless illuminating.

Living Wills and Advance Directives

Caring Connections (www.caringinfo.org) Here the National Hospice and Palliative Care Organization lists free resources to help family caregivers navigate a health crisis or end-of-life care, offers advice on planning strategies, and provides state-by-state living-will and advance-directive forms, all consistent with local legislation.

"CNH Fact-Sheet Series: Advance Directives/Living Wills" by the Compassionate Healthcare Network (www.chninternational.com/chnfact1.htm) In this article the CNH, a Canadian anti-euthanasia organization, lays out the argument against living wills and advance directives. The article, endorsed by the CNH, is quite a few years old (summer 1995), but it still resonates with alarmed compassion. British medical and legislative sources are cited. Perhaps it's worth reviewing before you sign your own living will.

Joint Centre for Bioethics, University of Toronto (www.jointcentreforbio ethics.ca) The Community Tools: Living Wills section is at www.joint centreforbioethics.ca/tools/livingwill.shtml. You'll have to sign in and accept some conditions before downloading any of several excellent living-will kits available here, including two that are specific to cancer and HIV. All are free and are well worth going through the sign-in process for—the JCB is world renowned for stimulating intelligent debate about health and ethics issues.

"Living Wills Ineffective, Say Medical/Legal Experts" by Donalee Moulton (www.lawyersweekly.ca/index.php?section=article&articleid=607) A growing number of Canadian legal and medical experts claim that living wills are ineffective because they ignore the fluid conditions of language and time. That's perhaps a nice way of saying that most living wills fail to keep pace with life changes. *The Lawyers Weekly*, where this article (dated January 25, 2008) appeared, is a Canadian newspaper for law professionals.

National Right to Life Committee (www.nrlc.org) The anti-euthanasia NRLC encourages its supporters to download a free copy of the group's Will to Live form instead of using a conventional living will. The NRLC argues that some physicians might choose to end life by withdrawing nutrition and that clear patient wishes are required.

Intensive Care

"ABC of Intensive Care: Recovery from Intensive Care" by Richard D. Griffiths and Christina Jones (www.bmj.com/cgi/content/full/319/7207/427) What happens after patients are discharged from intensive care? What's recovery like? This much-cited 1999 study prepares staff and families for post-ICU reactions that typically range from nightmares about being persecuted to a high level of physical debilitation due to severe muscle loss. *BMJ*, where this article (dated August 14, 1999) appeared, is published by a subsidiary of the British Medical Association.

Canadian Association of Critical Care Nurses (http://www.caccn.ca/en/pub lications/position_statements/ps2001.html) A well-reasoned position statement on withholding life support in intensive care, proposing conditions and practice standards for nurses who wrestle daily with the controversial issue.

Society of Critical Care Medicine (www.sccm.org) SCCM is an international organization with members from all the professions that staff an ICU. At the Web site click the MyICUCare icon at the top of the opening page to go to an informative section designed specifically for ICU patients and their families—a good primer on a hospital unit that seems frightening and mysterious.

Surgery

Keyhole Surgery Centre (www.keyholesurgerycentre.com.au/) Minimally invasive laparoscopy, often called keyhole surgery, is becoming more popular for minor procedures, and this Australian surgeon's Web site explains the technique better than most. Some graphic photographs here aren't for the queasy.

National Women's Health Resource Center (www.healthywomen.org) After reminding visitors to the Web site that most surgery patients are women, this nonprofit group offers excellent advice on preparation and recovery, as well as strategic information about all aspects of women's health. Though working in collaboration with leading health professionals, the NWHRC stresses that it is "independent of influence from external parties."

SpineUniverse (www.spineuniverse.com) Although the site specializes in the causes of back and neck pain and discusses the risks and rewards of surgical remedies and medications, it is also a good source for practical pain-management advice that doesn't always involve a scalpel or a bottle of pills.

Hospital Care

Hospital Compare (www.hospitalcompare.hhs.gov/) Sponsored by the U.S. Department of Health and Human Services, this site provides an easy way to give virtually any American hospital a quick check. Visitors are led through a stepped process that allows for up to three hospital comparisons, with variables like specialties and patient-satisfaction scores.

MedHunters.com (http://www.medhunters.com/articles/healthcareInCanada .html) While the debate over health-care rolls on in the United States, some American politicians favoring a more equitable system than is currently in place have taken a look at how Canada's public health care works. The article ("Healthcare in Canada") here at MedHunters, a site for health-job networking, is a quick primer from an American perspective. Notably, it points out that wait-times appear to lead the list of patient complaints on both sides of the border.

"Nurses' Report on Hospital Affairs in Five Countries" by Linda H. Aiken et al. (http://content.healthaffairs.org/cgi/content/full/20/3/43) *Health Affairs*, published by Project HOPE, is a professional journal specializing in health reform. This 1998–99 study is based on reports from 43,000 nurses in 711 hospitals in the United States, Canada, England, Scotland, and Germany. All spoke a common language of discouragement. Despite the age of the study, it remains current by drawing a direct link between deteriorating health care and cost cutting.

The Nursing Channel (www.nursingchannel.ca) Designed and managed by Toronto's huge University Health Network, this site serves up personal stories that define the best kind of nursing care. If you want to know more about the people who take daily care of your hospitalized loved one, this is a good place to start.

Hospice Care

Casey House (www.caseyhouse.com) Opened in 1988, North America's first freestanding hospice for people with HIV/AIDS now serves a population living longer than they used to with a still-incurable disease. Casey House was founded by the noted social activist June Callwood, who believed that everyone is entitled to die with dignity.

Hospice Foundation of America (www.hospicefoundation.org) The HFA is a nonprofit organization for families and professionals faced with someone's terminal illness. At the site you can find advice on choosing a hospice, research the process of dying, and get suggestions on coping with grief afterward. The home page includes a Locate a Hospice link.

International Association for Hospice and Palliative Care (www.hospice care.com) Founded by an oncologist who helped establish some of the first U.S. hospice programs, this group has the declared purpose of facilitating access to quality palliative and hospice care all over the world while working to ease the suffering associated with terminal or incurable illness.

St. Christopher's Hospice (www.stchristophers.org.uk) Cicely Saunders, considered the founder of the modern hospice movement, opened St. Christopher's Hospice in 1967. She died there in 2005.

Caregiver Support

Canadian Caregiver Coalition (www.ccc-ccan.ca) Signing in for Canadians as the "national voice for the needs and interests of family caregivers," this bilingual group provides current information on issues like caregiver burnout but also advocates for policy changes that acknowledge the huge social and financial contributions made by unpaid caregivers.

National Alliance for Caregiving (www.caregiving.org) A nonprofit U.S. coalition of various organizations that deal with family caregiving issues, the NAC explains its mission at this useful Web site: undertaking research studies, developing policies and programs, working to strengthen state and local caregiving groups, and representing the American caregiving community to the world.

National Family Caregivers Association (www.nfcacares.org) To educate, to support, to empower, to advocate are the four pillars of this nonprofit group. The NFCA estimates that there are fifty million caregivers in the United States. The group evolved from the friendship of two women who were looking after people suffering different illnesses but who found common ground in their caregiving needs and leaned on each other for support.

"Leading Advocate Proposes Guidelines to Create Systemic Support for Family Caregivers" by the United Hospital Fund (press release) (www .uhfnyc.org/press_release3159/press_release_show.htm?doc_id =424805) In case you're a busy caregiver with no time to pause and measure the personal cost of your work, browse this release from the New York–based nonprofit United Hospital Fund. It advocates the need for

encoding caregiver support and training into New York State policy, citing the burden carried by the state's estimated two million unpaid caregivers.

The Support Team Network (www.supportteam.org) Here's the buddy system at its best. This caregiver training and support center is a kind of
town hall for caregivers and would-be caregivers all over the United
States, a place where they can support one another with a mix of common
sense and smart strategies.

Miscellaneous

American Board of Medical Specialties (www.abms.org) At this Web site just
click the tabs that lead to board-endorsed consumer-education programs
(Newsroom, Events & Resources) and that let you check your specialist's
credentials (Is Your Doctor Certified?).

CarePages (www.carepages.com) With the best of intentions, friends will
sometimes nag obviously distracted families for progress reports on hospitalized loved ones. This outfit provides the means to easily create free
personal Web pages for patients. Many hospitals now encourage the practice.

Drugs.com (www.drugs.com) For a hit parade of sorts—a list of the top-sell-
ing drugs by brand name in the United States, see "Top 200 Drugs for
2007 by Sale" at www.drugs.com/top200.html. The ranking can provide
an unscientific clue to some of the most common ailments. For instance,
the most popular seller was Lipitor, a drug that lowers cholesterol. In second place was Nexium, which is used to reduce stomach acid. Both conditions have been linked to stress, and there's certainly a lot of that going
around. The Drugs.com home page gives you an A to Z Drug List.

Free Health, LLC (www.freehealth.com) Free Health says that its goal is
"solving the American Health Care Crisis one person at a time": by low-
ering the access-to-care bar with subsidized service discounts at a large
number of clinics and hospitals and by offering a basic health insurance
plan. The company, which launched its giveaway program in 2008, announced that it initially plans to hand out twelve billion dollars in health-
care benefits and millions of dollars in free surgeries. Participants present
a free card to their choice from a list of 285,000 health providers all over

the United States who have agreed to honor its various discounts. Is there a catch? None that is immediately obvious, but proceed cautiously anyway.

HealthWorld Online (www.healthy.net) Built around the image of a self-sustaining village, the site gives a global perspective on healthy living and self-managed care by citing both conventional and traditional health information. Though not for everyone, it does provide an interesting glimpse at alternative health options.

Medical Antiques (medicalantiques.com) Doug Arbittier, the physician who runs the site, shares pictures and information about his own collection, including surgical tools that look like medieval torture devices and elaborate china urns that once housed leeches for bloodletting. Take a fascinating jaunt into medicine's past that will make you glad all those devices are, well, in the past.

National Committee for Quality Assurance (www.ncqa.org/) Founded in 1990, NCQA is a prominent nonprofit organization dedicated to improving health-care quality by advocating for sound quality-measurement tools and programs that encourage the kind of accountability and transparency that lead directly to better care. But the group isn't driven solely by instructive methodology—it regularly cites and praises physicians as well as clinical programs for excellence.

"Preferences for a Patient-Centered Role Orientation" (http://springerlink. com/content/r4q8uuj1m75736q4/) All power to the patient? Not according to this 2004 study of 189 aging veterans undergoing care in an Iowa facility. Most did better when they simply followed doctors' orders and took no active role in their own care decisions. The study summarized here appeared in the *Annals of Behavioral Medicine* (February 2008); a complete copy can be downloaded in PDF form by clicking the appropriate icon on the Web page above.

RateMDs.com (www.ratemds.com) For doctor ratings and reviews, check out this site, which keeps a multinational scorecard. Reports on the performance of more than 150,000 doctors are provided by patients and families who claim personal experience with the practitioners. Most comments are positive, and a quick check may help you validate your own choice. But be cautious: There is no science here—merely personal opinion.

"Relating to Patients' Families" and "The Provider's Guide to Quality &
Culture" (http://erc.msh.org/mainpage.cfm?file=4.7.0.htm&module=
provider&language=English) and (http://erc.msh.org/mainpage.cfm?
file=1.0.htm&module=provider&language=English&ggroup=&m
group=) The first article helps care providers navigate through some of
the special needs of an emerging multiethnic population, including the
variable expectations of family presence, and the second offers advice
that is sensitive, compassionate, and reasonable. The site is the joint project of Management Sciences for Health and several other organizations
and departments and is funded in part by the U.S. Agency for International Development.

Index

Caregiver's Chart and Personal Journal
(Make as many photocopies as you need.)

Day 1   Date: _____

Patient Information

Name of Patient:

Age:

Family Doctor:

Blood Type:

Allergies:

Current Medications:

Preexisting Health Issues:

Next of Kin:

Principal Caregiver:

Designated Family Spokesperson (if different):

Important Phone Numbers for Family and Friends:

Available Dates and Times for Visiting/Care:

Patrick Conlon, *The Essential Hospital Handbook* (Yale University Press, 2009)

Hospital Information

Name of Hospital:
Address:

Date of Admission:

Reason for Admission:

Expected Length of Stay:

Actual Length of Stay:

Unit/Room Number:

Visiting Hours:

Treatment Plan:

Primary Doctor or Surgeon:

    Direct Line and/or Pager Number:

Unit Charge Nurse:

    Direct Line and/or Pager Number:

Nursing Station Direct Line:

Support Services Names and Contact Numbers:

Patrick Conlon, *The Essential Hospital Handbook* (Yale University Press, 2009)

Dietitian:

Pharmacist:

Physical Therapist (Physiotherapist):

Occupational Therapist:

Social Worker:

Chaplain:

Discharge Planner:

Discharge Plan

    Acceptable (yes/no):

    Issues to Be Discussed:

Tests Performed (blood work, X-rays, MRIs, CT [CAT] scans, etc.)

    In Room:

    Out of Room:

Results:

Patrick Conlon, *The Essential Hospital Handbook* (Yale University Press, 2009)

Procedures Performed (line installation, intubation, dressing changes, etc.):

  Patient's Reaction:

Medications Administered:

  Patient's Reaction:

Attending Doctor's Assessment:

Specialist Assessment (if applicable):

Dietary Changes:

Therapy—Physical and Occupational:

Therapy—Other (speech, etc.):

Grooming Tasks:

  Assigned to:

Bedside Assistance Provided by Caregiver:

Patient's Mood and Behavior:

Issues Raised with Care Staff:

  Outcome of Discussion:

Notes/Comments/Observations:

Patrick Conlon, *The Essential Hospital Handbook* (Yale University Press, 2009)

Caregiver's Chart and Personal Journal
(Make as many photocopies as you need.)

Day no. _____   Date: _____

    Tests Performed (blood work, X-rays, MRIs, CT scans, etc.)

        In Room:

        Out of Room:

    Results:

    Procedures Performed (line installation, intubation, dressing changes, etc.):

        Patient's Reaction:

    Medications Administered:

        Patient's Reaction:

    Attending Doctor's Assessment:

    Specialist Assessment (if applicable):

    Dietary Changes:

    Therapy—Physical and Occupational:

    Therapy—Other (speech, etc.):

Patrick Conlon, *The Essential Hospital Handbook* (Yale University Press, 2009)

Grooming Tasks:

Assigned to:

Bedside Assistance Provided by Caregiver:

Patient's Mood and Behavior:

Issues Raised with Care Staff:

Outcome of Discussion:

Notes/Comments/Observations:

Patrick Conlon, *The Essential Hospital Handbook* (Yale University Press, 2009)

Emergency Department Visit
(Make as many photocopies as you need.)

Name of Patient and Relationship:

Hospital:

Address:

Date and Time of Arrival:

Patient Is Alert/Aware? Confused? Uncomfortable? (If yes, rate as Mild, Moderate, or Severe.)

Purpose of Visit

    Injury (cause, if known):

    Illness (symptoms):

Seen by Physician (name and time):

Tests Ordered:

Results:

Consulting Physician or Surgeon (name and time):

Final Diagnosis:

Held for Observation?

Projected Length of Stay:

Patrick Conlon, *The Essential Hospital Handbook* (Yale University Press, 2009)

Care Plan

    Treated in ER?   How:

    Admitted to Hospital?   Why and Where?

When Discharged from ER:

Prescriptions to Be Filled:

Recommended Home Care:

Symptoms to Watch For:

Recommended Follow-up Action:

Bring:
   Proof of insurance (or health card)
   Name of family doctor and contact information
   List of patient's current medications (including herbal remedies and
      alternative therapies)
   List of patient's known allergies

Leave at Home:
   All of patient's valuables

Notes

Patrick Conlon, *The Essential Hospital Handbook* (Yale University Press, 2009)

Living Will Legal Consultation
(Make as many photocopies as you need.)

Name of Attorney:

Date and Time of Meeting:

Questions to Resolve before the Meeting

1. Do you want your organs donated?
   Yes   No   Yes, but under the following conditions:

2. If necessary, would you like to be resuscitated?
   Yes   No   Yes, but under the following conditions:

3. Do you want to be kept alive by life support?
   Yes   No   Yes, but under the following conditions:

4. Do you want all pain alleviated, even if it hastens death?
   Yes   No   Yes, but under the following conditions:

5. Would you like to be fed and hydrated through a tube?
   Yes   No   Yes, but under the following conditions:

6. Who will make all your medical decisions if you are unable (medical power of attorney)?
   Name:
   Address:
   Phone Number:

7. Where will copies of the living will be stored (for convenient access)?

Patrick Conlon, *The Essential Hospital Handbook* (Yale University Press, 2009)

Questions for Your Attorney

Are you ethically and morally comfortable preparing a legal document that could end my life?

Can the living will you prepare withstand court challenge in this (state/provincial) jurisdiction or in other jurisdictions outside your own?

Can it be updated easily and inexpensively as needs and preferences change?

Who needs to be notified about the existence of this living will?
Family:

Friends:

Family Physician:

Clergy:

Other:

Notes

Patrick Conlon, *The Essential Hospital Handbook* (Yale University Press, 2009)

Surgical Consultation
(Make as many photocopies as you need.)

Name of Patient and Relationship:

Date and Time of Meeting:

Place of Meeting:

Reason for Proposed Surgery:

Name of Surgeon:

Specialty:

Experience:

Recommended Procedure:

Open Surgery?
    Risks:
    Benefits:

Minimally invasive (Laparoscopic) Surgery?
    Risks:
    Benefits:

Review of Patient's Medical Records:

Examination of Patient:

Day Surgery:
    Estimated Length of Surgery:
    Estimated Time to Full Recovery:

Patrick Conlon, *The Essential Hospital Handbook* (Yale University Press, 2009)

In-Hospital Surgery:
    Estimated Length of Surgery:
    Estimated Length of Stay:
    Estimated Time to Full Recovery:

Anesthetic Required
    Local:
    Regional:
    General:

Predicted Level of Postoperative Discomfort
    Mild:
    Moderate:
    Significant:

Scheduled Date and Time of Preoperative Assessment:
    Place of Assessment:

Scheduled Date and Time of Surgery:
    Place of Surgery:

Bring:
    Proof of insurance or health card
    Name of referring physician and contact information
    List of patient's current medications (including herbal remedies
    and alternative therapies)
    List of patient's known allergies

Notes

Patrick Conlon, *The Essential Hospital Handbook* (Yale University Press, 2009)

Preoperative Assessment
(Make as many photocopies as you need.)

Location of Assessment Clinic:
    Phone Number:

Date and Time of Appointment:

Nurse in Charge of Assessment:

Blood Tests Required?
    Results:

Blood Pressure Reading Required?
    Results:

EKG Required?
    Results:

X-Rays Required?
    Results:

Results of Anesthetic Consultation:

Type of Anesthetic Proposed: Local   Regional   General

Scheduled Date, Time, and Place of Surgery:

Scheduled Date, Time, and Place of Follow-up with Surgeon:

Remember:
No food or drink (except water) after midnight before surgery
No alcohol 24 hours before surgery

Patrick Conlon, *The Essential Hospital Handbook* (Yale University Press, 2009)

Bring:

Proof of insurance

Name of family doctor and contact information

List of patient's current medications (including herbal remedies and alternative therapies)

List of patient's known medication allergies

Surgeon's notes and assessment requisition (if given to the patient to take to the assessment)

Notes

Questions for ICU Staff
(Make as many photocopies as you need.)

For the Nurses

Who are the doctors caring for my loved one?

Which doctor is in charge?

Is an intensivist involved in the care of my loved one?

Is there anything in the treatments planned for today that may be painful or uncomfortable?

If so, have medications been ordered to prevent the pain or discomfort?

If you're not in the room, how do I call for help?

How quickly should I expect someone to respond to the call?

How does my loved one go to the bathroom?

Can you explain to me what the doctor said?

Will you explain what all the tubes and equipment are and what they do?

What can I do to help?

What can I do to help my family and myself?

Should I bring anything from home?

Who can visit and when?

Patrick Conlon, *The Essential Hospital Handbook* (Yale University Press, 2009)

If I'm not in the hospital and something happens, how will you get in touch with me?

What happens if something urgent happens and I'm not available?

For the Doctors

What's wrong with my loved one?

Can it be cured?

How will this condition affect my loved one's quality of life?

What's the overall treatment plan?

When do you usually see a response to the treatment or therapy?

What changes will you be watching for as a response to the treatment or therapy?

What are the risks of the therapy and/or medications?

Is my loved one in any pain?

What's being done to ease my loved one's pain and fear?

How is nutrition provided?

Is my loved one receiving the medications to be taken at home?

Notes

Patrick Conlon, *The Essential Hospital Handbook* (Yale University Press, 2009)

Handy Hospital Information
(Make as many photocopies as you need.)

Name and Address of Hospital:

Key Hospital Phone Numbers:

    Patient:

    General Inquiries:

    Patient Inquiries:

    Patient Relations:

    Billing/Accounts Inquiries:

    Executive Offices:

Patient's Location (wing, floor, room number):

Name of Attending Physician:

    Pager Number:

Name of Charge Nurse:

    Nursing Station Direct Line:

Notes

Patrick Conlon, *The Essential Hospital Handbook* (Yale University Press, 2009)

Giving Updates to Family and Friends: Contact Information
(Make as many photocopies as you need.)

Name:

City/Town:

Relationship to Patient:

Home Number:

Work Number:

Cell Phone Number:

Pager Number:

Good Times to Call:

Notes (health issues, work/stress issues, etc.):

Name:

City/Town:

Relationship to Patient:

Home Number:

Work Number:

Cell Phone Number:

Pager Number:

Good Times to Call:

Notes (health issues, work/stress issues, etc.):

Patrick Conlon, *The Essential Hospital Handbook* (Yale University Press, 2009)

Caregiver Resources at the Hospital
(Make as many photocopies as you need.)

"I need a short break."
Location of Nearest Visitors' Lounge:

   Couch or Cot Available?
   TV or Music Available?
   Internet Connectivity Available?

Location of Nearest Book/Magazine Shop:

Location of Nearest Coffee Shop:

Location of Hospital Cafeteria: Hours Open:

Location of Shower Facilities:

Location of Hospital Chapel:

Location of Nearby Places to Stroll (landscaped hospital grounds, parks, shops):

"I need help resolving some questions and concerns."
Location of Patient Relations Office:
   Name of Person in Charge:

Name of Social Worker:
   Phone and Pager Numbers:

Name of Chaplain:
   Phone and Pager Numbers:

"Family are arriving, and we need a private place to talk."
Location of Nearest Family Room or Lounge:

Date and Time of Reservation:

Name and Title of Person Available to Answer Family's Questions:
   Phone and Pager Numbers:

Location of Nearby Hotel/Motel Accommodations:

Patrick Conlon, *The Essential Hospital Handbook* (Yale University Press, 2009)

Surrogate Caregivers: Who, What, When
(Make as many photocopies as you need.)

Name:

Phone Number:

Days and Times Available:

Willing to:
    Feed the Patient:
    Groom the Patient:
    Read to the Patient:
    Supply Music for the Patient:
    Assist in Bedside Tasks (moving the patient, etc.):
    Other:

Patient's Comments:

Staff Comments:

Patrick Conlon, *The Essential Hospital Handbook* (Yale University Press, 2009)

Agenda for a Family Meeting/Conference
(Make as many photocopies as you need.)

Name of Patient:

Unit and Room Number:

Date and Time of Meeting:

Place of Meeting:

Purpose
  Patient Progress Report:

  Complaint or Conflict (specify):

  Discharge Planning:

  Other (specify):

Family Members Present:

Staff Members Present:

Outcome/Result
  Action Proposed:

  Required Follow-up:

Notes:

Patrick Conlon, *The Essential Hospital Handbook* (Yale University Press, 2009)

Agenda for a Meeting to Plan Patient Discharge
(Make as many photocopies as you need.)

Name of Discharge Planner:

Date and Time of Meeting:

Place of Meeting:

Date of Anticipated Discharge:

Condition of Patient (caregiver's opinion):   Poor   Fair   Good
  In the caregiver's opinion, is the patient ready for discharge?

  If no, state reasons:

What an Effective and Comprehensive Discharge Plan Should Include

1. The continuing care services the patient will need, including medical treatments, medical transportation, and homemaker services.

2. Detailed information about the services that have been arranged.

3. Names, addresses, and phone numbers of the service providers.

4. A schedule outlining when at-home nursing or rehabilitation services will begin.

Patrick Conlon, *The Essential Hospital Handbook* (Yale University Press, 2009)

5. Medications that the patient will need and clear instructions for their use.

6. Information about special diets and treatments, including dietary restrictions, if any.

7. The detailed schedule for any of the patient's follow-up medical appointments.

8. Advice on what to monitor at home, including fever or any bleeding, and who to call in the event of an emergency.

9. A detailed explanation of the process of appealing a discharge decision, including staff members to contact and forms to complete.

Notes

Patrick Conlon, *The Essential Hospital Handbook* (Yale University Press, 2009)

Home Preparation Checklist

(Make as many photocopies as you need.)

Safety Check

A ramp to the front door to accommodate a wheelchair or a walker?

A clear path through each room, with no rugs or raised room dividers to trip over and no slippery floors?

Furniture rearranged to ease navigation?

Handrails to help move from one room to another?

A raised toilet seat for easier sitting?

Grab bars near the toilet and bathtub for safety in standing and sitting?

Non-skid mats on the bathroom floor and in the bathtub to prevent slipping and falling?

Nightlights for safety in moving around at night?

Working smoke alarms and fire extinguishers throughout the home?

Emergency numbers—fire, hospital, 911—and contact numbers in a convenient location?

Special Equipment Check

A hospital bed or other special type of bed?

Walker? Cane? Wheelchair?

Bedside commode?

Lift?

Oxygen?

Mobility Check

Is a ramp needed on exterior stairs?

Will a wheelchair fit through doorways?

Is it easy to walk or move from room to room without running into furniture?

Communication Check

Get a cordless speaker phone with speed dial, making it possible to call for emergency help with one push of a button and avoid compromising the safety of your loved one?

Patrick Conlon, *The Essential Hospital Handbook* (Yale University Press, 2009)

Get a phone with a large digital display for easy reading, plus a ring and voice enhancer, if your loved one has a vision or hearing problem?

Get a fully charged cell phone if you and your loved one will be spending time outside the home?

Install a medical or home alert system making it possible to summon help with the push of a button if you will occasionally leave your loved one alone?

Get an intercom or baby monitor in order to listen to your loved one when you are in another room?

Get a hand bell or buzzer that your loved one can use to ring for help?

Notes

Patrick Conlon, *The Essential Hospital Handbook* (Yale University Press, 2009)

Presurgery Medications Checklist
(Make as many photocopies as you need.)

Prior to Surgery, Patients Can Take:

    Heart medications
    Antireflux medications (Prilosec, Nexium, Protonix)
    Seizure medications (anticonvulsants)
    Anti-hypertensives (blood pressure medications)
    Bronchodilators (inhalers and medications for the lungs)
    Birth control pills
    Steroids (prednisone)
    Immunosuppressants
    Thyroid replacement (Synthroid)
    Anti-Parkinson medications
    COX-2 antagonists (Vioxx, Celebrex)
    Opiates (without aspirin; Tylenol #3, Vicodin, fentanyl, etc.)

Prior to Surgery, Patients *Should Not* Take:

    Chewable antacids (Tums, Rolaids, etc.)
    Diuretics (water pills, furosemide, hydrochlorothiazide)
    Insulin
    Oral hypoglycemics (Glucophage, Avandia, Actos, DiaBeta,
        Micronase, Glucotrol, Amaryl)
    Aspirin (and compounds that contain ASA)
    Nonsteroidal anti-inflammatory drugs (ibuprofen, Motrin, Advil,
        Mobic, Orudis, etc.)
    Potassium
    Weight reduction agents
    Vitamins
    Herbal supplements

Notes

Patrick Conlon, *The Essential Hospital Handbook* (Yale University Press, 2009)

Medical/Surgical Follow-up Appointments
(Make as many photocopies as you need.)

Name of Physician or Surgeon:

Address:

Phone Number:

Pager:

Date and Time of Appointment:

Special Instructions:

Notes:

Name of Physician or Surgeon:

Address:

Phone Number:

Pager:

Date and Time of Appointment:

Special Instructions:

Notes:

Patrick Conlon, *The Essential Hospital Handbook* (Yale University Press, 2009)

Hospital Complaints Process
(Make as many photocopies as you need.)

Complaint Specifics
　　Date of Incident:
　　Time of Incident:
　　Place of Incident:
Communication (lack of information, misunderstanding, or inappropriate communication):
Patient Care (medical error; personal or clinical treatment of patient):
Patient Services (food, hospital room, sanitation, or infection-control lapses):
Hospital Policy (visiting hours, other policies, surgery cancelled because of lack of beds):
Other (health provider conduct, treatment of caregiver, treatment of other family members or visitors, etc.):

Steps to Take
1. If the scope of the complaint is limited to the hospital unit housing the patient, discuss the complaint with:
　　Charge Nurse (name):
　　　　Date of Conversation:
　　Satisfactory Resolution?　　Yes　　No　　Explain:
If not satisfied, contact:
　　Unit/Program Manager (name):
　　　　Date of Conversation:
　　Satisfactory Resolution?　　Yes　　No　　Explain:
2. If the complaint could affect others or has not been resolved, register a written complaint with the senior executive responsible for patient relations (name):
3. Outline your concerns clearly, using the 5 W's: who, when, where, what (or how), and why.
4. Copy the hospital CEO and the unit/program manager on all correspondence.

Patrick Conlon, *The Essential Hospital Handbook* (Yale University Press, 2009)

What to Expect

1. A letter or phone call acknowledging your complaint.
2. An investigation involving all parties, including interviews with the patient, family, and staff and perhaps a review of the patient's medical chart.
3. A report that may include the following recommendations:

    Making a patient relations specialist available for ongoing consultation with the family

    Providing feedback to the staff involved and providing training if necessary

    Outlining specific actions for improvement

4. Follow-up by the management to confirm compliance with all the recommendations.

Patrick Conlon, *The Essential Hospital Handbook* (Yale University Press, 2009)

Questions When Choosing a Hospice
(Make as many photocopies as you need.)

Patient's Needs and Wishes
How do the hospice staff, working with the patient and loved ones, honor the patient's wishes?

Family Involvement and Support
Are family caregivers given the information and training they need to care for the patient at home?

What services does the hospice offer to help the patient and loved ones deal with grief and loss?

Is respite care (relief for the caregiver) available?

Are loved ones told what to expect in the dying process and what happens after the patient's death?

What bereavement services are available after the patient dies?

Physician and Staff
What is the role of the patient's physician once hospice care begins?

How will the hospice physician oversee the patient's care and work with the patient's doctor?

How many patients does each hospice staff member care for?

Volunteers
What services do volunteers offer?

What screening and type of training do hospice volunteers receive?

Comfort and Pain Management
Do the hospice staff regularly discuss and routinely evaluate pain control and symptom management with patients and families?

Do the hospice staff respond immediately to requests for additional pain medication?

What specialty or expanded programs does the hospice offer?

How does the hospice meet the spiritual and emotional needs of the patient and the family?

Patrick Conlon, *The Essential Hospital Handbook* (Yale University Press, 2009)

After-Hours Care

How quickly do hospice staff respond to after-hours emergencies?
Are a chaplain and a social worker available after hours? Are others?
How are calls and visits handled when death occurs?

Various Care Settings

How does the hospice provide services for residents in nursing homes
and other such care settings?
How does the hospice work with hospitals and other facilities during
the course of the patient's stay?
What will happen if care cannot be managed at home?

Quality of Care

What credentials do the hospice staff have? Do they have special cre-
dentials in their specialties?
Is the hospice program certified and licensed?
What other kind of accreditation or certification does the hospice pro-
gram have? How about its staff?
What measures does the hospice take to ensure quality?

Paying for Hospice Care

Are all of the costs of hospice care covered by the patient's health insurance?
What services will the patient have to pay for out of pocket? Are any services provided at no charge?

Patrick Conlon, *The Essential Hospital Handbook* (Yale University Press, 2009)